THE COMPLETE CASTOR OIL BIBLE

3 in 1 Experience the Ultimate Journey in Natural Wellness with Recipes and Proven Strategies for Optimal Health, Radiant Beauty, and an EcoFriendly Lifestyle

Waverly Christie

TABLE OF CONTENTS

BOOK 1: "CASTOR OIL ESSENTIALS: HEALTH REMEDIES AND HEALING SECRETS"

CHAPTER 1: THE FUNDAMENTALS OF CASTOR OIL

Welcome to the world of castor oil—a journey that transcends ancient tradition and touches the core of today's natural wellness practices. Often enveloped in mystery and surrounded by tales of healing, castor oil remains one of nature's most versatile and nurturing gifts. Exploring its benefits and uses is not just about understanding a plant oil; it's about rediscovering a path to holistic health that our ancestors trod long before us.

Derived from the seeds of the castor plant, Ricinus communis, which thrives in the warm regions of the world, castor oil has a rich history that dates back to ancient Egypt. It was a treasured potion, believed to be used by Cleopatra herself for the brilliance it bestowed upon the skin and eyes. Its journey through time saw its adoption by varied cultures, each finding new ways to harness its extensive properties.

The process of extracting castor oil is as fascinating as its history. Through a method known as cold pressing, the oil retains most of its healing attributes, ensuring that every drop carries the potent benefits that were revered by our forebears. This extraction method emphasizes the oil's purity, a critical factor as we delve into its health and beauty applications.

The distinct properties of castor oil—ranging from its antiinflammatory effects to its ability to enhance moisture retention in skin and hair—stem from its rich chemical composition. Rich in ricinoleic acid, a rare fatty acid, castor oil offers benefits that are broad and deepreaching. From soothing inflamed skin to improving hair health, it operates not merely as a remedy but as a foundation for nurturing one's health.

As we unfold the layers of castor oil's uses in the following sections, keep in mind that this humble oil is not just a substance but a bridge to an improved state of wellbeing. Whether you seek solutions for health ailments or desires for beauty enhancements, understanding the fundamentals of castior oil is the essential first step on this remarkable journey.

1.1 HISTORY AND ORIGIN

The tapestry of castor oil's history is woven with colorful threads stretching back to the dawn of civilization. Its story is a captivating chronicle of mystery, medicine, and myriad uses that have evolved over millennia.

Long before the modern conveniences of today's beauty and health products, there was castor oil—a potent elixir valued by ancient cultures for its remarkable therapeutic properties.

The journey of castor oil begins in the ancient lands of Egypt, around 4000 B.C., where it was initially cultivated. Historical records, including Ebers Papyrus—one of the oldest preserved medical documents—detail the use of castor oil for lamps and as a natural remedy to protect the eyes from irritation. The oil was not only a household staple but also part of spiritual practices, where it was believed to purify and cleanse both the body and spirit.

As trade routes expanded, so too did the knowledge and use of castor oil. It found its way into the hands of the Greeks and Romans, who admired its laxative and purgative properties. The famed physician Dioscorides extolled castor oil as an ointment for troubling skin ailments and wounds, writing at length about its virtues in his medical texts. His Roman counterpart, Pliny the Elder, also documented the oil's considerable benefits in his encyclopedic work, *Natural History*, emphasizing its role in burning lamps and anointing the body.

The castor plant, from which the oil is derived, is known botanically as *Ricinus communis*. It is a fastgrowing, perennial shrub that can attain astonishing growth in a single season, suggesting a kind of vigor and potency that is mirrored in the properties of its oil. The seeds, which are primarily composed of the triglyceride ricinolein, are pressed to extract the oil—a method that has remained largely unchanged over centuries. It is noteworthy, however, that these same seeds contain ricin, a highly toxic substance, making the process of oil extraction a careful art that ensures the removal of hazardous components while preserving the beneficial ones.

Transitioning into the medieval age and later into the Renaissance, castor oil's reputation flourished across continents. It was a panacea of sorts in folk medicine, prescribed for nearly everything—from inducing labor to healing inflamed tissues. African and MiddleEastern communities especially revered the oil for its hydrating and healing properties in harsh, arid climates.

In the 18th and 19th centuries, as explorers ventured into new territories, castor oil plants were introduced to the Americas. The oil gained a prominent position as a treatment for colic and other digestive issues in children. It was also during this era that industrial uses of castic oil began to surface. The burgeoning automotive industry found a resource in castor oil for lubricating engines, a testament to its versatility and resilience under high temperatures.

Fast forward to the 20th century, and we observe the integration of castor oil into modern pharmaceuticals and cosmetics. Its emollient and antiinflammatory properties made it a favorite ingredient in skin creams, hair conditioners, and even drugs designed to deliver specific medication effectively.

Its ability to penetrate deep into the skin has seen castor oil embraced by the beauty industry, valued equally for its ability to moisturize and its capacity to carry other therapeutic agents deep beneath the skin's surface.

However, the usefulness of castor oil extends beyond its physical applications. The environmental consciousness of the 21st century has revived interest in sustainable and biodegradable substances, with castor oil emerging as an ecofriendly alternative in various applications, including biofuels and biodegradable plastics. This aligns beautifully with a renewed global commitment to sustainable agriculture, as *Ricinus communis* is remarkably hardy, requires minimal pest control, and thrives on marginal lands, making it a low impact crop.

Perhaps most profoundly, the history and evolution of castor oil reflect a broader narrative about humanity's relationship with nature—how we continually return to the natural world for solutions to our most pressing challenges. From a simple seed to a symbol of wellness and sustainability, castor oil's journey through time is as rich and deep as the oil itself. It serves as a reminder of the legacy left by our ancestors, who recognized the value of what nature provided and learned how to harness its power for their wellbeing.

As we explore the contemporary uses and benefits of castor oil, let us appreciate the depth of history it carries and the breadth of potential it holds for the future. Whether in medicine, beauty, industry, or agriculture, castor oil continues to offer invaluable contributions to health and wellness, echoing the ancient wisdom that has permeated cultures around the globe.

1.2 EXTRACTION AND PROCESSING TECHNIQUES

Delving into the realm of castor oil extraction and processing unveils a fascinating blend of traditional wisdom and modern technology. Essential to unlocking the potent benefits of castor oil, these techniques are not just about obtaining an oil but ensuring that it retains its rich therapeutic properties and is safe for use. Perfecting the art and science of extracting castor oil involves sophisticated methods that have been honed over centuries, adapting to the changing times and technologies yet rooted in ageold practices.

The castor plant, *Ricinus communis*, provides the seeds from which the oil is derived. Each seed is a small but mighty repository of oil, typically making up 4060% of its weight. The initial step in the extraction process is the harvesting of these seeds, primarily grown in India, Brazil, and China, areas known for their favorable climatic conditions that nurture the growth of this hardy plant. Handpicked for quality, the seeds are then cleaned to remove dirt and debris, ensuring that only the best go into the oilmaking process.

Historically, the traditional method of extraction involved cold pressing, a mechanical process that crushes the seeds without external heat. This method is favored for its ability to maintain the integrity of the oil's chemical structure, preserving its nutritional and medicinal properties.

The cold press method operates on the principle of pressure, where castor seeds are gradually compressed in a controlled environment to extract the oil. The lack of heat ensures that delicate compounds within the oil, like ricinoleic acid, are not destroyed, thus keeping the oil's healing qualities intact.

Once the oil is extracted, it undergoes a purification process to remove any impurities and the hazardous ricin, a potent toxin naturally present in the seeds. Ricin does not integrate into the oil during cold pressing, primarily settling in the leftover seed cake. Yet, to ensure safety and purity, manufacturers perform thorough filtration and sometimes employ methods like heat treatment or solvent extraction to cleanse any residual traces.

Solvent extraction offers an alternative to cold pressing, often used in largescale production due to its efficiency. This method involves using a chemical solvent, usually hexane, to dissolve the oil from the seed mash. Although it yields higher amounts of oil, solvent extraction can affect the natural qualities of the oil due to the chemicals used and the higher temperatures applied. Once extracted, the oil is refined to remove the solvent traces, a step essential for ensuring the product's safety and quality.

Another innovative approach in the realm of castor oil production is the use of hybrid techniques, where mechanical pressing is combined with solvent extraction to boost the yield and purity. This method capitalizes on the efficiency of both worlds—starting with a mechanical press to obtain a primary extract followed by solvent treatment to recover additional oil from the leftover biomass. Regardless of the method, quality control is paramount. Each batch of castor oil undergoes rigorous testing to ensure it meets the industry standards of purity and efficacy. Parameters like color, acidity, moisture content, and fatty acid composition are meticulously monitored. The packaging also plays a crucial role in preserving the quality of oil; hence, inert materials that do not react with the oil or contribute to its degradation are chosen for storage.

Environmental considerations are also central to the extraction and processing of castor oil. Sustainable practices are increasingly employed across the spectrum from the cultivation of castor plants to the final handling and disposal of byproducts. Efficient waste management systems are in place to deal with the biomass residue, often repurposed as organic fertilizer or animal feed, thus promoting a zerowaste approach.

In understanding these methods, we gain not only a deeper appreciation of the labor and ingenuity involved in bringing this remarkable oil to our shelves but also the complexities of ensuring that each drop of castor oil can deliver the maximum health and beauty benefits. The convergence of technology and tradition in castor oil production is a testament to humanity's ongoing commitment to harnessing nature's gifts while respecting and preserving its integrity.

As we embrace castor oil's offerings, let us also acknowledge the sophisticated dance of science and nature that brings such natural remedies into our daily lives.

1.3 VARIETIES AND THEIR UNIQUE PROPERTIES

Within the verdant realms where *Ricinus communis* unfolds its glossy, palmate leaves lies a spectrum of diversity that might surprise even those already familiar with castor oil's benefits. This oil, renowned for its healing attributes, is extracted from the seeds of castor plants, which vary intriguingly across different geographical and climatic zones. These variations give rise to distinct types of castor oil, each possessing unique properties and uses that enrich our understanding and application of this ancient wellness tool.

The core types of castor oil are primarily categorized based on the method of extraction, which directly influences their attributes and suitability for various applications. The most common is the coldpressed castor oil, celebrated for preserving the integrity of essential nutrients and enzymes. This oil is extracted under pressure without the use of heat, ensuring that the critical beneficial compounds, like ricinoleic acid, remain intact. Coldpressed castor oil is typically clear or slightly yellowish in color and is considered the highest quality grade for medicinal and cosmetic applications due to its purity and nutrient richness.

In contrast, Jamaican Black Castor Oil (JBCO) offers a darker, ashier hue, a reflection of the roasting process that the seeds undergo before oil extraction. This technique is traditional to Jamaica and involves roasting the castor seeds, grinding them, and then boiling them to extract the oil. The result is a product that retains some of the ashes from the roasted seeds, believed to contribute to its highly regarded efficacy in promoting hair growth and rejuvenating skin. JBCO is especially venerated for its ability to restore moisture and enhance the softness of hair and skin, making it a staple in beauty regimens around the world.

Another variant, the hydrogenated castor oil, known technically as castor wax, is produced by the addition of hydrogen to pure castor oil under controlled conditions. This process transforms the oil into a waxy substance, which is solid at room temperature. Castor wax is predominantly used in cosmetics, polishes, and varnishes, providing durability and shine.

The pharmaceutical grade of castor oil is characterized by its exceptional purity and sterility, making it suitable for use in medical applications. This oil is often employed in formulations that require a high degree of precision and safety, including topical ointments and as a carrier for medicinal compounds.

Beyond these common types, new varieties of castor oil continue to emerge, driven by continual research and development efforts aimed at maximizing its therapeutic and industrial potentials. Innovations in genetic modification and cultivation practices have also led to the development of specialized castor plants that can thrive in lessthanideal soil conditions, expanding the geographical reach of castor oil production.

The diverse chemical composition of castor oil largely defines its therapeutic properties. Ricinoleic acid, an omega9 fatty acid unique to castor oil, accounts for about 90% of its fatty acid content and is largely responsible for its antiinflammatory, antimicrobial, and moisturizing properties. Moreover, castor oil contains other beneficial salts and esters that contribute to its antioxidant, antifungal, and antibacterial benefits.

These varying types of castor oil can be chosen and used depending on the specific needs and outcomes desired. For instance, while coldpressed castor oil is ideal for health and beauty applications due to its purity and nutrient content, Jamaican Black Castor Oil might be preferred for hair care solutions due to its potency in promoting hair growth and scalp health.

With such versatility, castor oil not only illustrates the complexities of nature but also demonstrates the adaptability of natural products to meet the evolving needs of human health and beauty. Each type of castor oil holds a narrative that reflects its origin, from the fields where the castor plants are harvested to the traditional or modern methods employed in its extraction.

Understanding these variations enriches our appreciation of castor oil and enhances our ability to use it effectively, bridging ancient natural wisdom with modern lifestyle needs. As we integrate these diverse types of castor oil into our daily routines, we not only benefit from its profound healing properties but also participate in a legacy of natural health that spans cultures and generations.

CHAPTER 2: CASTOR OIL FOR INTERNAL HEALTH

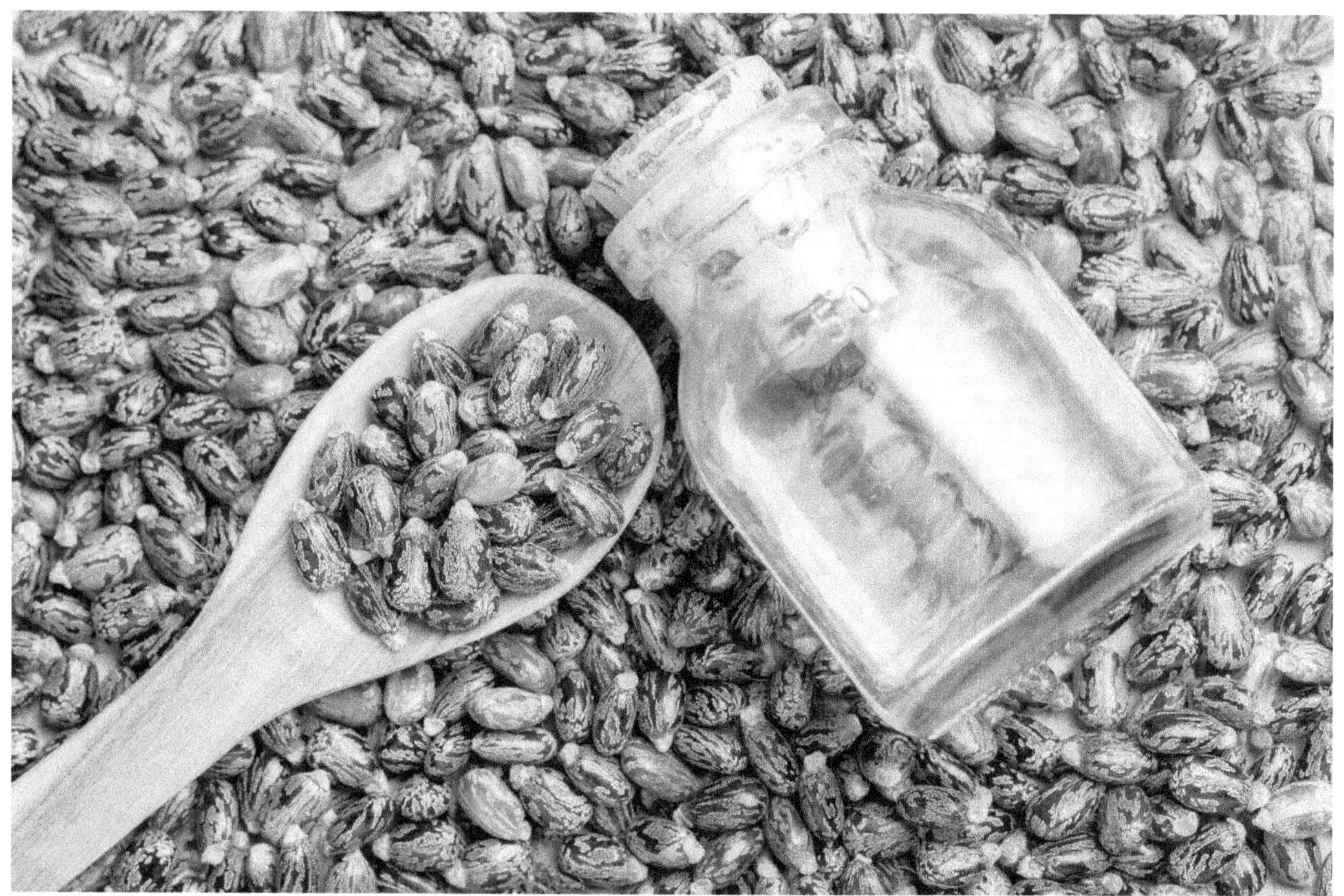

Within the vast expanse of natural remedies, castor oil emerges not only as a balm for the external body but as a potent elixir for revitalizing our internal systems. Its rich history, steeped in centuries of traditional use, only scratches the surface of its deep reservoir of health benefits. In this chapter, we delve into the remarkable capabilities of castor oil to enhance digestive wellness, boost our natural immune defenses, and support the body's detoxification processes.

Imagine a gentle, soothing companion travelling through your digestive tract, easing inflammation, and nurturing the mucosal linings. Castor oil acts not just as a lubricant but as a healer that soothes on contact and aids in efficient digestion and nutrient absorption. This golden oil has been a trusty ally against common digestive ailments, offering a gentle yet effective solution where harsh chemical treatments may not.

Turning to immunity—a cornerstone of good health—castor oil offers its fatty acids as knights in shining armor. These molecules naturally bolster the body's defenses, turning the simple act of consuming or applying castor oil into a strengthening ritual for our immune system. In this way, casty oil helps create a robust barrier against seasonal illnesses and common health threats.

Moreover, in our increasingly toxic world, the gentle detoxifying properties of castor oil provide a beacon of hope.

It supports the liver, our body's primary detox organ, in its neverending task of cleansing the blood and other tissues. This oil's unique ability to stimulate circulation aids in removing toxins at a cellular level, promoting a purified, energized body environment.

By integrating castor oil into your daily health regimen, you're not just using a natural product; you're embracing a centuriesold tradition of holistic health. This chapter will guide you through understanding how this powerful oil supports internal balance and wellness, ensuring that your journey towards optimal health is as enriching as it is natural. So, let us embark on this journey together, exploring the internal health miracles of castor oil, your natural ally in achieving a vibrant, balanced life.

2.1 ENHANCING DIGESTIVE WELLNESS

In our journey with castor oil, we find its influences on our health are as deep as they are profound. One of its most significant contributions lies in its ability to enhance digestive wellness. Throughout the ages, traditional practitioners spanning diverse cultures have recognized the efficacy of castair oil in soothing and supporting the digestive system. Today, modern advocates and holistic health practitioners continue to celebrate its benefits, integrating this timeless elixir into contemporary wellness regimens.

The relation between digestion and overall health is inextricably linked—a welloiled digestive system is the bedrock of vitality. It is here that castor oil plays its pivotal role.

When ingested, castor oil acts as a stimulant laxative, encouraging the muscles of the intestine to move, thus facilitating easier elimination. This gentle encouragement helps in maintaining regular bowel movements which is foundational to digestive health.

Castor oil's benefits extend beyond mere stimulation of bowel movements. Its unique composition, rich in ricinoleic acid, provides soothing relief to the intestinal lining. This specific fatty acid binds to receptors on the smooth muscle cells of the intestinal walls, causing contractions that aid in the movement of food through the intestials. It is particularly beneficial in cases of constipation, a common ailment affecting a significant portion of the population, often leading to discomfort and lethargy. By ensuring regular bowel movements, castor oil helps in the effective elimination of waste and toxins, thus enhancing nutrient absorption, and potentially alleviating symptoms of bloating and discomfort.

Moreover, this remarkable oil has been known to exhibit antiinflammatory properties, which can be tremendously beneficial in managing and alleviating symptoms of inflammatory conditions such as Irritable Bowel Syndrome (IBS) and Crohn's disease.

These conditions, characterized by inflammation in the digestive tract, can cause severe discomfort and a range of symptoms including abdominal pain, cramping, and severe constipation. Regular use of castor oil can help to moderate these inflammatory responses, providing relief and improving quality of life for those affected.

Perhaps one of the less discussed but equally important roles of castor oil in digestive health is its impact on gut microbiota—the vast community of microorganisms that reside in our digestive tract. Emerging research suggests that the antimicrobial properties of castor oil may help in balancing gut flora, thus contributing to a healthier intestinal environment. A balanced gut microbiota is crucial for proper digestion, synthesis of vital nutrients, and an overall strong immune system.

Beyond its physical health benefits, the influence of castor oil on digestive wellness also spreads to emotional and mental health. The gut is often referred to as the "second brain," with a vast network of neurons that communicate directly with the brain. Maintaining digestive health with natural aids like castor oil not only ensures physical comfort but can also enhance mood and cognitive function, underlining the holistic impact of a wellsupported digestive system.

Incorporating castor oil into your lifestyle for enhanced digestive wellness does not require grand gestures. A simple, moderate approach can be equally effective. However, it is crucial to proceed with knowledge and caution.

Castor oil, while beneficial, is potent, and its dosage and frequency of use should be carefully managed. Overuse may lead to adverse effects such/not as diarrhea and dehydration, which can disrupt electrolyte balance and overall health.

To safely integrate castor oil into your regimen for digestive wellness, it is recommended to start with small doses, observing how your body responds before gradually increasing the amount, if necessary. It's also advisable to consult with a health professional or a knowledgeable practitioner in natural medicine who can provide guidance tailored to your specific health needs.

Users should ensure the purity and quality of the castor oil purchased, as these factors significantly influence the oil's effectiveness and safety. Organic, coldpressed castor oil is typically recommended due to its quality and minimal processing, which helps in retaining most of its beneficial properties.

In conclusion, the journey of enhancing digestive wellness with castor oil is a testament to the power of natural remedies in supporting and revitalizing our internal systems. By fostering a better understanding of its properties and mindful integration into our lives, castor oil can serve as a loyal and effective ally in our ongoing quest for health and vitality.

Through such natural solutions, we honor not only the wisdom of traditional practices but also the incredible capacity of our bodies to heal and thrive in harmony with nature.

2.2 BOOSTING IMMUNITY NATURALLY

In the realm of natural health remedies, castor oil holds a storied place as a robust promoter of wellness, not least of which pertains to boosting immunity—a critical aspect of maintaining health in an age where modern lifestyles often compromise our natural defenses. The journey to understanding how castor oil contributes to immune enhancement is not only fascinating but also provides us with actionable insight into leading healthier, more resilient lives.

Castor oil's immuneboosting properties can be traced back to its chemical composition, rich in ricinoleic acid—a rare and highly effective compound known for its antiinflammatory and antibacterial benefits. When castor oil is used, it not only helps fight infection through direct action but also boosts the body's own defensive mechanisms. This duality of direct and indirect action makes castor oil a particularly potent tool in the natural health arsenal.

The immune system functions as the body's natural defense mechanism against infections, diseases, and various external invaders. In this intricate system, balance is paramount. An overactive immune system can lead to allergies and autoimmune diseases, while an underactive one can render the body vulnerable to infections.

Here, castor oil's role is to help modulate the immune system's response, aiding in a balanced immune reaction that effectively wards off illnesses without overreacting dangerously.

Ricinoleic acid acts by supporting the lymphatic system, which is a critical component of the immune system.

The lymphatic system, comprising lymph nodes and flowing lymphatic fluids, is essential for the transport of white blood cells throughout the body and for detoxifying the internal environment. Castor oil applied topically can penetrate the skin and stimulate the lymphatic system, enhancing the flow of lymphatic fluids. This stimulation supports the body's ability to detoxify, circulate nutrients, and rouse white blood cells to defense posts where they are most needed. Improved lymphatic circulation means that the body becomes more efficient at detecting and responding to pathogens or threats, thus enhancing overall immunity.

The detoxifying properties of castor oil also contribute significantly to its ability to boost immunity. By helping remove toxins and waste materials from the body, castor oil ensures that the immune system does not become overwhelmed. This clearing of potential threats lowers the chance of developing an inflammatory response, which can tax the immune system and lead to chronic health issues if persistently triggered.

Aside from its physical health benefits, castor oil can impact psychological wellbeing, which in turn influences immune strength. Stress is wellknown as a suppressor of immune function. The soothing properties of castor oil can reduce stress, thereby indirectly supporting immune health. When used as part of a massage or in a warm bath, castor oil can help relax the mind and reduce physiological manifestations of stress, creating a more conducive environment for the immune system to function effectively.

In integrating castor oil into your routine for immune health, it is vital to consider the method of application. Although primarily used topically, due to concerns about its potent laxative effects when ingested, understanding the correct topical application is key to maximizing its immuneboosting potential. Applying it to areas abundant in lymph nodes, such as around the abdomen, neck, and underarms, can be particularly effective. Compresses soaked in castor oil, placed on the skin, can also be a potent method of transdermal absorption, stimulating both circulation and lymphatic drainage.

However, the use of castor oil, particularly in new users, should be approached with care. Due diligence in selecting highquality, coldpressed, and preferably organic castor oil is essential to avoid contaminants or additives that can undermine its health benefits. Additionally, as with all potent remedies, starting with small amounts and observing the body's response is critical. Consulting with a health professional knowledgeable in natural medicinal practices can provide personalized guidance and ensure safety.

Ultimately, castor oil denotes a confluence of history, science, and holistic health practice—a trifecta that offers a powerhouse of benefits, especially in enhancing immune function.

By embracing the responsible, informed use of this traditional remedy, we equip our bodies with a natural ally capable of safeguarding and enriching our health. Thus, the narrative of castor oil is not merely one of historical use but a continuing story of beneficial integration into modern wellness practices, supporting the body's innate strengths and promoting a balanced, healthy immune response. Through this lens, we see not just an oil, but a legacy of wellness that enriches our present and empowers our future.

2.3 DETOXIFICATION AND CLEANSING

Our bodies are remarkable systems that continuously process and eliminate toxins through organs like the liver, kidneys, and skin. However, the modern lifestyle, which often includes processed foods, environmental pollutants, and stress, can place an extraordinary burden on these detox mechanisms. Enter castor oil, a traditional remedy revered not just for its healing capabilities but also for its profound detoxifying properties.

Castor oil's role in detoxification and cleansing is rooted deeply in both historical practice and modern holistic health. It is derived from the seeds of the Ricinus communis plant and has been used therapeutically across the world for centuries. Central to castor oil's detoxifying prowess is its ability to support the body's vital organs responsible for purification and elimination of substances that can harm the body if allowed to accumulate.

The primary component of castor oil, ricinoleic acid, plays a pivotal role by its stimulating effect on the lymphatic system. The lymphatic system is a crucial part of the immune system, comprising a network of tissues and organs that help rid the body of toxins, waste, and other unwanted materials. The proper functioning of the lymphatic system is essential for detoxification, yet it often lacks its own pumping mechanism, relying instead on body movement and muscular contraction to propel fluids through its vessels.

When applied topically, castor oil has been shown to enhance the flow of lymph, helping to increase the rate at which toxins are cleansed from tissues and assisting in the reduction of swelling, inflammation, and pain. Castor oil compresses—applied to different parts of the body such as the abdomen, liver area, or swollen joints—can be particularly effective in stimulating lymphatic drainage and promoting healing from within.

Furthermore, the detoxifying power of castor oil extends to the liver, the body's primary detoxification organ. The liver filters and detoxifies blood, breaks down hormones, and helps digest fat. Castor oil packs applied to the liver area can help enhance liver function, potentially aiding in the detoxification process and improving liver health overall.

This application is believed to facilitate the liver's ability to eliminate toxins, sometimes enhancing regeneration of cells and reducing inflammation.

The benefits of castor oil in detoxification also include its support for digestive health, as mentioned previously. By improving bowel regularity, castor oil helps prevent the reabsorption of toxins from the gut. A properly functioning digestive system is pivotal in preventing toxins and byproducts from leaking back into the body, thus supporting overall detox processes.

Although less direct, the holistic impact of castor oil on stress reduction and immune function also contributes to detoxification. Stress can severely impede the body's natural ability to detoxify because it diverts the body's energy away from the detoxification processes towards managing stress. By promoting relaxation and improving sleep—effects attributed to the soothing properties of castor oil—this natural remedy helps maintain an environment where the body's detox systems can function optimally.

Despite these substantial benefits, the use of castor oil, particularly for detoxification purposes, should be approached with mindfulness and respect for individual health conditions.

Quality of the oil is crucial; organic, coldpressed castor oil is preferred for topical use due to its purity and retained beneficial properties. Furthermore, for those new to using castor oil, it is advisable to incorporate it gradually and observe how the body responds. Consulting with a healthcare provider knowledgeable in natural remedies can provide additional guidance tailored to your individual needs.

Importantly, while castor oil is a potent aid in detoxification, it complements rather than replaces the foundational elements of health, such as a balanced diet, adequate hydration, regular exercise, and proper sleep. These factors all contribute to the body's innate ability to cleanse itself and should not be overlooked in the pursuit of a detoxification regimen.

Through the lens of holistic health, castor oil emerges not only as a therapeutic agent but as a symbol of the gentle strength inherent in nature's offerings. Its use invites us to reconnect with traditional wisdom while embracing the benefits of contemporary holistic health practices, affirming that sometimes, the most profound healing comes from the purest sources.

Chapter 3: Pain Relief and AntiInflammatory Uses

In our journey through the profound versatility of castor oil, we arrive at a chapter dedicated to one of its most cherished benefits: natural pain relief and antiinflammatory properties. It is here, amidst the crowded shelves of modern pharmaceuticals, that casty oil stands quietly potent, harkening back to ancient wisdom while embracing the embrace of contemporary science.

Imagine the plight of Ellen, a school teacher in her midforties, who first came to me weary with the burden of arthritis in her joints. Each morning presented a painful battle, each movement a measure of endurance. Ellen was skeptical, her experiences with conventional medicine providing only temporary relief shadowed by unwelcome side effects. Yet, within weeks of integrating castor oil applications into her routine, she reported a significant ease in her symptoms. For Ellen, castor oil wasn't just a treatment but a gateway to reclaiming joy in everyday activities—gardening, playing with her grandchildren, and even simple tasks like opening jars or writing on the blackboard.

This transformative potential of castor oil is not confined to anecdotal testimony but is underpinned by its biochemical composition. Rich in ricinoleic acid, a rare fatty acid, castor oil naturally possesses antiinflammatory and analgesic properties. When applied topically, it penetrates deeply, combating inflammation at the source, soothing sore muscles, and alleviating joint pain. Moreover, its therapeutic prowess extends to headache relief—where a gentle temple massage with diluted castor oil can diffuse the throbbing pain of a migraine, allowing tranquility to seep back into one's day.

As we explore the myriad ways to utilize castor oil for pain relief, from arthritis and joint pain to muscle aches and headaches, it is essential to approach each method with a mindfulness of its origins and effects. The subsequent sections will guide you through specific recipes and application techniques that are not only effective but also a testament to the resilience and adaptability of nature's solutions. In embracing these methods, we do more than treat symptoms— we engage in a holistic ritual of healing, honoring our bodies and the earth from which this golden elixir flows.

3.1 Treating Arthritis and Joint Pain

Arthritis and joint pain, ailments as ancient as human history, have meandered through civilizations, leaving traces of their presence in countless lives. Today, they persist as prominent disruptors of comfort and mobility, nudging many towards a relentless search for relief.

Among the multitude of therapeutic agents, castor oil shines with particular brilliance—a remedy espoused not only in the annals of tradition but also increasingly validated by the discerning lens of modern science.

The story of castor oil as a panacea for joint pain begins in the lush landscapes of ancient Egypt, where it was more than just a medicine—it was a symbol of protection and healing. Fast forward to today, its relevance has only deepened, particularly given the contemporary push towards more natural and sustainable health practices.

Arthritis, in its many guises, primarily involves the inflammation of joints, leading to pain, stiffness, and a diminished range of motion. This inflammation can be the body's immune response gone awry or simply the wear and tear of daily life. Castor oil enters the scene as a combatant of inflammation due to its high content of ricinoleic acid—a remarkable fatty acid that not only fights inflammation but also deeply penetrates the skin to soothe affected areas.

The method of applying castor oil for arthritis and joint pain is delightfully simple yet profoundly effective. Surrounding this practice is a tapestry of stories, such as that of Martin, a carpenter who had been wrestling with the swelling and stiffness in his knees for years. For Martin, retirement seemed the only option, a thought that brought a premature sense of defeat. However, upon integrating castor oil packs into his nightly routine, he noticed an improvement that pills had never provided. The warmth of the oil combined with its therapeutic properties brought a significant reduction in pain, enabling him to move freely and embrace his craft once again.

Castor oil's mechanism involves not just the direct soothing effect of its application but also a broader impact on the body's lymphatic system. The lymphatic system, a critical part of the immune system, helps in removing toxins and waste from the body. When castor oil is applied, it stimulates lymphatic circulation, which in turn reduces inflammation and accelerates the removal of cellularrelated waste products in the joints. This dual action—direct antiinflammatory effect and enhancement of lymphatic function—is what can make castor oil a particularly potent remedy for arthritis.

To tap into this ancient yet effective remedy, users often employ castor oil packs—a method that involves soaking a piece of wool or cotton flannel in castor oil, placing it on the affected area, and covering it with a heat source, such as a heating pad. This process enhances the oil's penetration and increases its efficacy by promoting the absorption of ricinoleic acid through the pores of the skin.

Moreover, the use of castor oil for arthritis is aligned with a holistic approach to health. It involves not just addressing the symptoms of arthritis but fostering an environment of overall wellness.

For instance, its application is often paired with mindfulness practices, gentle exercise, and a balanced diet, creating a comprehensive strategy against the ailments.

Discussions in the health community about natural remedies often swing between skepticism and advocacy. However, the narrative around castor oil is strengthened by both historical precedence and emerging scientific research. Studies suggest that its antiinflammatory properties can be as effective as certain overthecounter pharmaceuticals, presenting it as a possible alternative for those inclined towards natural remedies.

It is also important to consider the broader implications of choosing natural remedies like castor oil. In an era where environmental concerns are at the forefront, the sustainable nature of castor oil—readily biodegradable and derived from a renewable resource—makes it a steward of both personal and planetary health.

Yet, while the benefits are compelling, the path of natural remedies requires patience and persistence. The effects of castor oil, for instance, may not be as immediately dramatic as pharmaceutical alternatives, but its advantages are found in its gentle approach and cumulative benefits.

In the constellation of natural remedies available for arthritis and joint pain, castora oil is but one star, albeit a bright one. Its application is a testament to the enduring wisdom of nature, offering a blend of tradition and modernity that resonates with today's holistic health paradigm. As more individuals like Martin rediscover these ancient remedies, the narrative of natural healing continues to unfold, woven into the fabric of modern medicinal practices, promising relief and renewed mobility to those who venture into its warm embrace.

3.2 SOOTHING MUSCLE ACHES AND STRAINS

In the realm of physical exertion, whether through sports, labor, or the simple act of navigating daily life, muscle aches and strains are frequent visitors. These types of discomforts whisper (or sometimes shout) the needs of our bodies, emphasizing the fine line between pushing our limits and nurturing our wellbeing. Here, in the soothing embrace of nature's remedies, castor oil emerges as a poignant solution, a custodian of relief that blends ancient tradition with modern holistic practices.

For those unfamiliar with its scientific prowess, castor oil, derived from the seeds of the Ricinus communis plant, has established its efficacy primarily through its high concentration of ricinoleic acid. This unique compound is revered not only for its potent antiinflammatory properties but also for its ability to act as an analgesic, providing relief from pain.

When muscles are overworked or improperly used, they signal distress through swelling and pain, processes that are intimately tied to inflammation. Ricinoleic acid works by inhibiting the release of inflammationtriggering compounds in the body, offering a natural, gentle respite from discomfort.

Consider the story of Julia, an avid gardener whose passion for her craft often left her with sore muscles at the end of a fulfilling day in her sprawling vegetable and flower beds. Traditional pain relief methods provided her little solace, often accompanied by undesirable side effects. Turning to castor oil as a holistic alternative, she found not just relief but also a new ritual in her gardening lifestyle. By applying a castor oil pack to her sore areas, she noticed a profound easing of tension and a quicker recovery time, which enabled her to pursue her gardening with renewed vigor and minimal discomfort.

In this context, the application of castor oil goes beyond mere symptom management. It invites a holistic view of body care, encouraging users to engage actively with their wellbeing through natural means. Applying castor oil, particularly through massages or packs, not only delivers the oil's intrinsic benefits but also enhances blood flow to the affected area. Improved circulation is an essential element in muscle recovery, helping to flush out inflammationcausing toxins and speeding up the healing process.

The method of applying castot oil can be quite therapeutic. The act of massaging the oil into the skin is a moment of connection between mind and body, a nurturing practice that honors the body's need for care and attention. Through gentle, circular motions, the muscles are warmed and relaxed, and the deep penetration of the oil is facilitated, enhancing its effectiveness and providing a muchneeded respite from pain.

In discussions among both health practitioners and those who turn to natural remedies for relief, the versatility of castor oil often comes to the forefront. Its use in treating muscle aches is supported by both anecdotal evidence and an increasing body of scientific research that highlights its role in reducing inflammation and pain, making it a viable alternative to chemicalbased creams and ointments.

The growing popularity of castor oil in muscle care also speaks to a broader societal shift towards more sustainable and healthconscious living. As people become more attuned to the origins and impacts of the products they use, the appeal of a naturally derived, minimally processed substance like castor oil continues to grow. Its production, which requires minimal chemical intervention, aligns with the ethos of environmental stewardship and sustainability, marking it as a choice that benefits both personal health and the health of the planet.

Even as its benefits are celebrated, it is crucial for users to approach the use of castor oil with mindfulness. Understanding one's body's responses and respecting its limits is paramount. While castor oil is generally considered safe, its application should be adjusted to individual needs and circumstances, including the specific area of pain and the severity of the strain.

As this narrative unfolds, the story of castor oil in soothing muscle aches and strains is not just about alleviating pain but about embracing a holistic, responsive approach to body care. In its essence, it is about empowering individuals to take charge of their health, to listen intently to their bodies, and to respond with natural, effective remedies that honor both their immediate needs and their longterm wellbeing. For those who incorporate castor oil into their muscle care routine, it is not just a remedy but a ritual, a testament to the power of nature's pharmacy and the profound connection between the natural world and the human body.

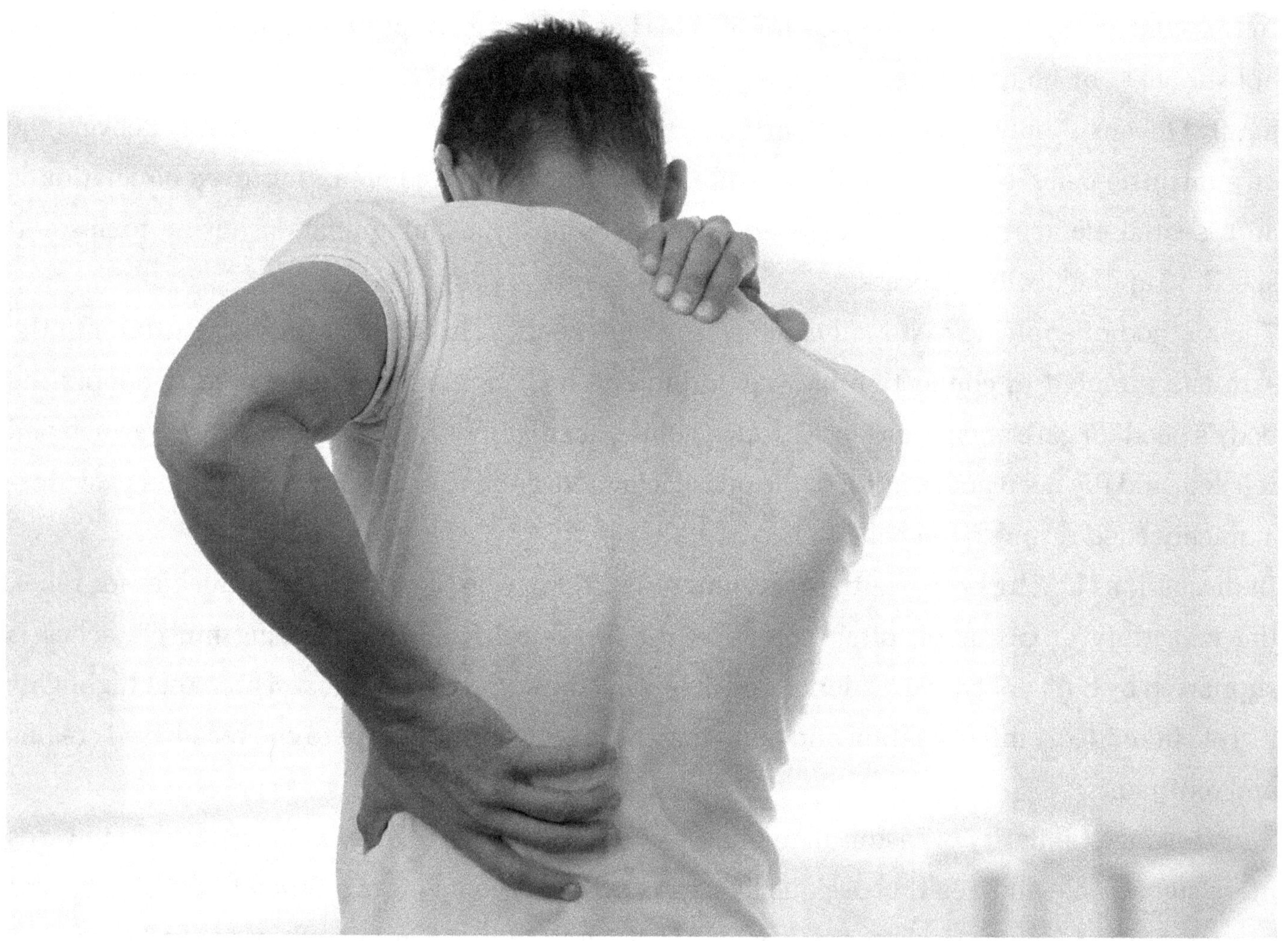

3.3 REMEDIES FOR HEADACHES AND MIGRAINES

In the intricate ballet of daily life, headaches and migraines often appear as unwelcome interludes, disrupting rhythm and harmony. Among the diverse palette of remedies available, castor oil emerges as a soothing balm, a timehonored salve with roots deep in the annals of herbal medicine.

Its efficacy in addressing such cerebral discomforts makes it not just a remedy but a ritual of relief and recovery, guiding individuals back to their optimal states of wellbeing.

Headaches, ranging from the mundane tensiontype to the debilitating throes of migraines, are often symptomatic of underlying physiological or psychological imbalances such as stress, dehydration, or sleep disturbances. Here, castor oil steps into the limelight not merely as an analgesic but as an antiinflammatory agent capable of addressing the root causes of these pain episodes. Its high concentration of ricinoleic acid serves as the key player—an agent that when massaged into the scalp, can dilate blood vessels and improve blood flow, thus easing the tightness and pain associated with headaches.

Consider a typical scenario involving Emily, a graphic designer whose profession chains her to the rigors of tight deadlines and long hours before glaring screens. The frequent throbs of tension headaches began to encroach upon her productivity and peace. The turning point came when she incorporated castor oil into her routine, applying a light film to her temples and the nape of her neck during breaks. Over time, Emily found that these applications not only lessened the severity of her headaches but also imbued a sense of calm, allowing her to navigate her demanding profession with renewed poise.

The process of applying castor oil for headaches and migraines is intuitive and simple, enabling its integration into daily routines.

By lightly massaging the oil onto the scalp, temples, or neck, one can initiate its penetrating action, which not only alleviates the pain but also relaxes the mind. This dual action makes it particularly effective during those times when psychological stress manifests as physical pain.

Moreover, the inclusion of castor oil as a remedy for headaches aligns closely with holistic principles, emphasizing prevention and the nurturing of overall health. This alignment speaks to those who are increasingly seeking out natural and proactive approaches to health management, wary of the quick fixes offered by conventional medicine, which often come with a barrage of side effects.

The benefits of castor oil extend beyond the immediate easing of pain, promoting a systemic balance that can preempt future episodes. For instance, its use might enhance lymphatic drainage, an oftenoverlooked factor in the accumulation of toxins that can contribute to headaches and migraines. By facilitating the removal of these toxins from around the head and neck area, castor oil helps maintain a clearer pathway for nerve signals and blood circulation, key components in the prevention of headache disorders.

The narrative of castor oil in the management of headaches and migraines draws on its larger story within natural medicine—a story of rejuvenation, resilience, and return to balance. As individuals like Emily continue to share their experiences, they weave castor oil more tightly into the fabric of communal knowledge, underscoring its worth not only as a treatment but also as a testament to the wisdom inherent in natural remedies.

Yet, it's crucial for users to approach their use of castor oil with mindfulness, recognizing that each individual's experience of pain is unique. The exact method of application and frequency can be tailored to suit individual needs and responses, ensuring that this ancient remedy can find its place in the modern repertoire of therapeutic practices.

In today's fastpaced world, where quick solutions often overshadow sustainable wellness practices, castor oil offers a bridge back to simplicity and balance. Its use in treating headaches and migraines is not just about relief but is part of a broader conversation about health autonomy and the preventive power of nature's own medicine cabinet.

In conclusion, the journey through the pain of headaches and migraines with castor oil is not merely about alleviating symptoms but about embracing a lifestyle that values slow medicine and comprehensive health. It's a testament to the potent capabilities of natural remedies, serving as a gentle reminder of our own capacity to heal and thrive in rhythm with the natural world.

CHAPTER 4: RESPIRATORY HEALTH AND WELLNESS

Amidst the whirlwind of modern life, with its smogfilled cities and relentless demands, maintaining respiratory health has become a cornerstone for a thriving existence. It's no wonder that a return to more natural, triedandtrue remedies like castor oil is not just a trend, but a necessity for many.

For centuries, castor oil has been a silent guardian and a remedy, extracted from the humble castor seed and its rich, healing essence. This chapter delves into the therapeutic uses of castor oil in bolstering respiratory wellness, a vital component of holistic health. As the seasons change, bringing with them the common cold and allergy flareups, the versatility of castor oil offers more than just relief; it offers a promise of a healthier life.

Imagine a typical cold winter morning. The air is biting, and amid the hustle of the daily grind, you feel the onset of a scratchy throat and stuffed nose. Instead of reaching for overthecounter cold remedies that often bring unwanted side effects, consider the natural alternative. A simple inhalation of steam infused with castorous compounds can open breathing passages, reduce inflammation, and soothe the respiratory system.

But how does this ancient remedy stand up to the rigors of modern ailments like sinusitis and allergies? Through testimonials and scientific backing, we explore how the unique properties of castor oil can be harnessed to not only manage symptoms but enhance overall respiratory health. From homemade vapor rubs to warm compresses, this chapter will guide you through a variety of applications, ensuring that you are wellequipped to handle the respiratory challenges that life may throw your way.

By integrating castor oil into your wellness routine, you are choosing a path that respects both tradition and science, blending them beautifully to create solutions that are as nurturing as they are effective. Embrace the potency of castor oil and breathe easier knowing that your respiratory health is in good hands. Join me on this journey to discover the breath of relief offered by nature's own elixir.

4.1 ALLEVIATING COMMON COLD SYMPTOMS

As the leaves turn and the air chills, it is not uncommon to hear the familiar sniffles and coughs that signal the onset of the common cold. A nuisance at best and debilitating at worst, the common cold has a way of making its presence felt. While modern medicine offers a plenitude of synthetic remedies, the gentle, yet effective nature of castor oil presents a timehonored solution worth considering.

Castor oil, with its thick, viscous consistency and a faint, distinctive smell, has been used as a healing elixir for centuries. Its application spans diverse ailments, but its role in alleviating the symptoms of the common cold is particularly noteworthy. Through its antiinflammatory, antibacterial, and antiviral properties, castor oil works to soothe and reduce the symptoms that make colds such an inconvenience.

The initial invasion of a cold virus typically brings with it a sore throat. The linoleic acid found in castor oil serves as a potent antiinflammatory agent, helping to soothe throat irritation. When applied as part of a throat compress or used in steam inhalation, it can provide substantial relief. The warmth of the compress coupled with the penetrating properties of the oil works to reduce throat swelling and alleviate pain, making it easier to handle the daily tasks that don't pause with our health.

Following the sore throat, nasal congestion often ensues, turning breathing from a subconscious action to a conscious effort. Here, too, castor oil can play a pivotal role. Its efficacy in reducing inflammation can be utilized to relieve swollen nasal passages, enhancing airflow and facilitating easier breathing. Inhaling steam that carries the microscopic particles of this oil can help loosen the mucus buildup, and when the vapor penetrates the airways, it can also help inhibit further microbial growth in the nasal passages and respiratory tract.

Furthermore, the common cold often brings with it a general feeling of discomfort and malaise. Castor oil's component, ricinoleic acid, not only fights inflammation but also has analgesic properties which can help reduce general body aches associated with the cold. Applying a castor oil pack over the abdomen or on sore joints can help reduce pain transmission, providing a comforting relief.

Beyond direct applications, castor oil's holistic influence on immune system fortification should not be overlooked. By supporting lymphatic drainage, it helps in detoxifying the body—a major boon when it's fighting an infection. This detoxifying effect not only helps to shorten the duration of a cold but also enhances overall vitality, which can be particularly depleted during such times.

It's also worth noting the benefits of integrating castor oil into your regular health regimen as a preventive measure. Regular use of castor oil, be it in the form of packs, massages, or in aromatherapy, can help bolster the body's defenses against the common cold. By maintaining a body environment that balances detoxification with immune support, castor oil helps prepare the body to fend off infections more efficiently.

Lastly, although much of castor oil's acclaim springs from anecdotal evidence backed by centuries of traditional uses, a growing body of scientific reviews and studies begin to paint a picture of its mechanisms and effectiveness. These studies, while still in earlier stages, complement the historical narrative of castor oil as a remedy and provide a foundation for its continued use today. In conclusion, when the common cold strikes, casting an eye towards the humble castor seed might provide not just relief, but a gentle, natural pathway to recovery. By understanding and utilizing the multifaceted properties of castor oil, one can manage and mitigate the symptoms of the common cold, turning what is often a weeklong ordeal into a more manageable, and perhaps shorter, recovery period. While it is no panacea, castor oil's role in soothing, healing, and enhancing body resilience stands out as a testament to nature's bounty.

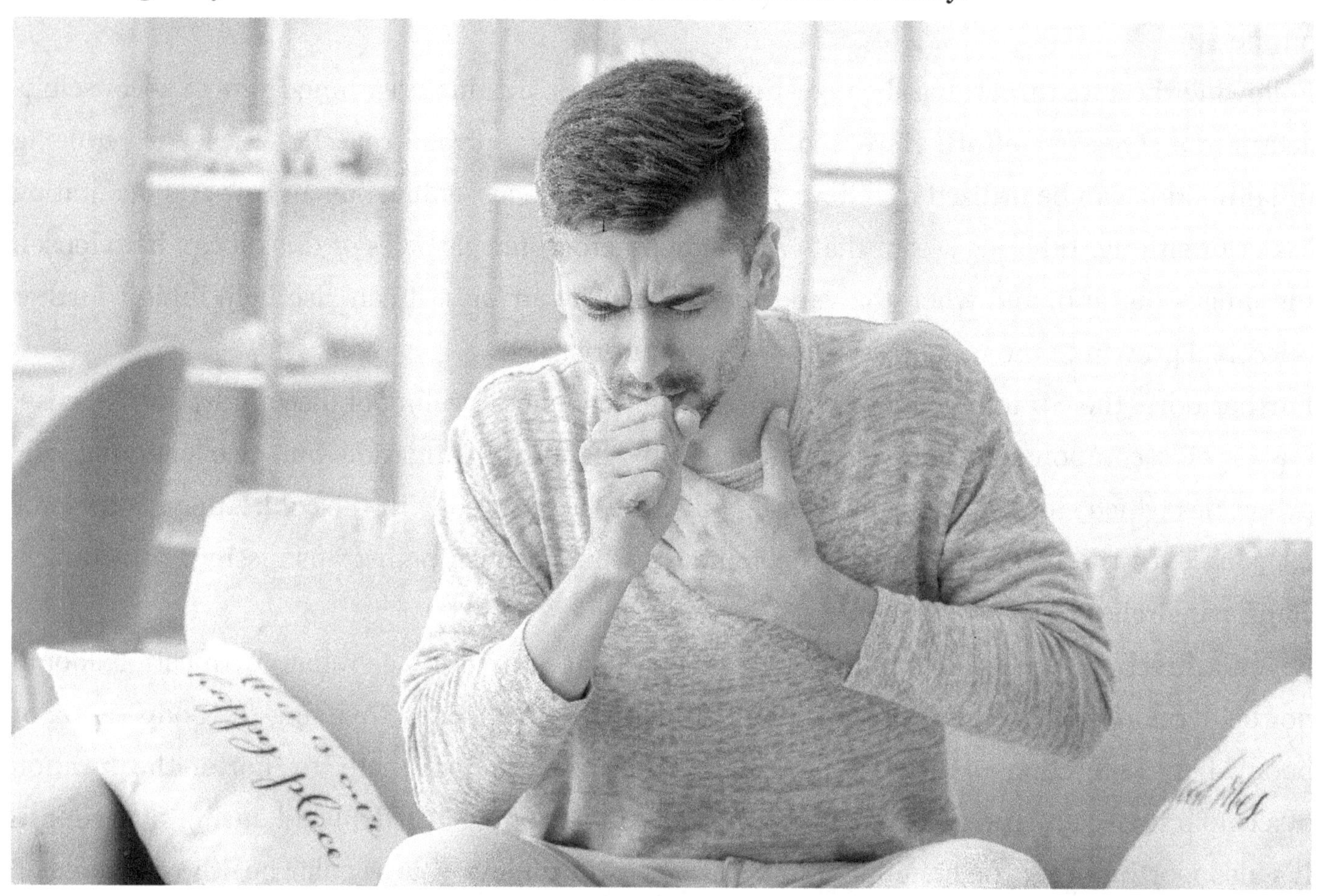

4.2 NATURAL TREATMENTS FOR SINUSITIS

In the labyrinth of natural remedies and ancient wisdom, castor oil emerges as a trusted ally against the persistent discomfort of sinusitis. This condition, characterized by the inflammation of the sinuses, results in symptoms that disrupt daily life: from painful pressure in the facial region to a blocked nose, and oftentimes, an overarching malaise. The journey through these winding passages of discomfort can be arduous, but with castor oil, a path to relief is palpable.

Sinusitis often results from either an infection or an allergic reaction, leading to swollen nasal passages that hinder normal breathing and drainage. Conventional treatments typically range from antibiotics to surgery, depending on severity, but many seek gentler, less invasive alternatives. Here, the ageold virtues of castor oil are rekindled, offering soothing relief through its unique medicinal properties.

The primary component of castor oil, ricinoleic acid, exhibits powerful antiinflammatory properties which play a crucial role in reducing the swelling of mucous membranes along the sinus cavities. This reduction in inflammation can significantly ease the pain and improve airflow, allowing the sinuses to drain naturally and relieve builtup pressure.

Moreover, castor oil is known for its antimicrobial properties. When dealing with sinusitis caused by bacterial infections, these properties become particularly advantageous, helping to fight the bacteria within the sinus cavities while nurturing the nasal tissues back to health.

For those suffering from chronic sinusitis, the journey often includes frequent doctor visits and a procession of different medications. Integrating castor oil into daily routines provides a form of empowerment—a way to take control and actively manage the condition with a natural solution. Applying warm castor oil externally over the sinus areas can help enhance blood circulation to the affected regions, promoting healing and offering comfort.

But the benefits of castor oil go beyond mere symptom relief. The oil's ability to support the immune system is of paramount importance. Sinusitis, particularly when chronic, can be a telling sign of an underlying imbalance or weakness within the immune system. By fortifying the body's defenses, castan oil helps address not only the current inflammation but also works to prevent future occurrences.

One of the lesserknown aspects of castor oil is its role in stimulating the lymphatic system. Proper functioning of the lymphatic system is essential for the removal of toxins and waste from the body. When this system is efficient, the body's capacity to fend off infections, including those affecting the sinuses, is considerably enhanced.

Moving from theory to practice, consider the application of a castor oil pack over the sinus areas. This method involves soaking a piece of wool flannel in castor oil, placing it over the face while avoiding direct contact with the eyes, and applying heat for enhanced penetration. Such a treatment can turn into a soothing ritual, providing a moment of peace in the hustle of everyday life, while the therapeutic properties of the oil work to ease the sinuses.

For anyone considering the use of castor oil for sinusitis, it's important to remember that while castor oil can provide considerable relief, it is not a cureall.

In cases of severe or acute sinusitis, consulting with a healthcare provider is recommended. However, for ongoing maintenance and prevention, as well as mild to moderate cases, castor oil stands as a beacon of relief.

Through narrativerich scenes like the one where an elder recalls how his grandmother would treat his childhood sinus episodes with nothing but a bottle of castor oil and a warm cloth, to the more recent accounts of individuals finding relief in their battle with chronic sinusitis, the tales abound. This connection through time enriches the narrative of castor oil, emphasizing not just its efficacy but also its role in human health and heritage.

Thus, as we navigate the complexities of modern health dilemmas, the simplicity and efficacy of natural remedies like castor oil provide a comforting solution. With its deeprooted history and proven benefits, castor oil for sinusitis is not merely a treatment, but a testament to the enduring power of nature's own medicine cabinet.

4.3 MANAGING ALLERGIES WITH CASTOR OIL

In a world where allergies seem as common as the dandelions popping up in springtime lawns, finding effective, natural remedies is akin to discovering a hidden garden of relief. Among these, castor oil emerges not as a miracle cure, but as a potent ally in the ongoing battle against allergic reactions, especially those that afflict the respiratory system.

Allergies, which affect millions globally, manifest through an array of symptoms including sneezing, congestion, and itchy, watery eyes; all of which can transform beautiful spring days into periods of dread. The root cause? An immune system response to harmless substances like pollen or dust which it mistakenly identifies as threats. Here, castor oil enters the narrative, offering soothing relief through its extraordinary properties.

Primarily known for its antiinflammatory benefits, castor oil addresses the swollen nasal passages and airways that can exacerbate allergic symptoms. By applying the oil to the chest or incorporating it in vapor form through steam inhalation, individuals can experience eased breathing as the antiinflammatory agents work to reduce swelling and irritation.

Additionally, the rich antioxidative nature of castor oil plays a crucial role in fortifying the body's defenses. Antioxidants help in quelling the oxidative stress that might complicate allergies. In this way, castor oil doesn't just fight the symptoms but enriches the body's immune response against ongoing allergenic attacks.

One of the less highlighted, yet significant, properties of castor oil is its ability to support lymphatic drainage.

A functioning lymphatic system efficiently removes toxins and other unwanted substances from the body, which can be particularly beneficial for allergy sufferers, whose systems are often overwhelmed with histamines and other chemicals during allergic reactions. By enhancing the flow of lymphatic fluids, castor oil helps ensure that these irritants are removed more efficiently, potentially reducing the severity and duration of allergic responses.

Moreover, the calming effect of castor oil can also extend to the skin, which might suffer from allergic reactions like hives or eczema. The application of castor oil directly to affected areas can hydrate and heal the skin, providing relief from itchiness and irritation, which, while peripheral to respiratory symptoms, often accompany allergic episodes.

For individuals looking towards integrating castor oil into their allergy management regimen, it's vital to consider it part of a broader lifestyle approach. While castor oil can provide symptomatic relief, managing allergies effectively often includes avoiding known allergens, maintaining a clean home environment, and possibly using air purifiers to reduce the presence of airborne allergens. The stories that underscore the efficacy of castor oil are many and varied. Consider an anecdote about a young woman, burdened by seasonal allergies, who discovered relief through nightly castor oil packs, claiming reduced morning congestion and fewer allergic reactions during high pollen periods. Or tales from parents who've mixed a few drops of castor oil with other natural oils to create soothing chest rubs for children, helping them sleep peacefully despite high allergen levels.

While scientific research into the full spectrum of castor oil's benefits, particularly in relation to allergies, continues to grow, the empirical evidence provided by centuries of traditional use is substantial. Users worldwide praise its natural, less invasive approach to symptom management, valuing both its efficacy and the peace of mind that comes from using a nonpharmaceutical remedy.

In essence, managing allergies with castor oil is about embracing an ancient, yet still relevant, approach to health—one that respects the body's natural rhythms and seeks to restore balance and wellbeing. Like a gentle guardian, castor oil offers a protective embrace to those suffering from the overzealous responses of their own immune systems. As each season unfolds, with its particular allergens and challenges, turning to castor oil can be a wise and comforting strategy in the quest for relief and health.

CHAPTER 5: COMPREHENSIVE HEALING RECIPES

As we delve into the heart of our journey with castor oil, we uncover its profound ability not just to soothe but to restore. Chapter 5, "Comprehensive Healing Recipes," is crafted to transform your kitchen into a sanctuary of health. Through whispers of the past, where wise elders concocted elixirs of wellness, we draw inspiration; yet, our approach marries tradition with modern insight, offering you remedies that are both timeless and tested.

Imagine standing in your kitchen, the earthy scent of castor oil blending with other natural ingredients. Here, you're not just preparing remedies; you're brewing a revolution of wellness. Each recipe in this chapter is a thread in the fabric of holistic health, designed to address everything from the quiet rumblings of an upset stomach to the sharp twinges of inflammation. With each stir and mix, you're crafting your own narrative of health, one spoonful at a time.

Think about Laura, a mother of two, balancing work and family while battling chronic arthritis. Traditional medications had offered little relief and brought along numerous side effects. Frustrated and weary, she turned to one of our recipes—a simple castor oil blend infused with herbs. Within weeks, Laura noticed a decrease in pain and an improvement in her mobility. Her mornings transformed from painstaking to hopeful. Laura's story is not just about alleviating physical pain but about reclaiming joy and activity.

As you explore the recipes in this chapter, remember that each concoction is more than just a mixture; it's a testament to the power of nature and your own healing journey. From digestive health to respiratory relief, the solutions we offer are designed to empower you, giving you the tools to nurture your body naturally.

In embracing these recipes, you embrace a part of a broader community seeking sustainable, effective health solutions. Let the alchemy of castor oil guide you to not only manage symptoms but to thrive in a rhythm of wellness that sings to the tune of nature's simplicity and purity.

CASTOR OIL GINGER ELIXIR

Ingr:

- 1 Tbls castor oil
- 1 tsp freshly grated ginger
- 1 C. warm water
- 1 Tbls fresh lemon juice
- 1 tsp honey

Proc:

- Mix castor oil with warm water
- Add freshly grated ginger, lemon juice, and honey
- Stir well until completely blended
- Drink on an empty stomach

Benefits:

- Aids in digestion and reduces bloating
- Enhances detoxification
- Provides antiinflammatory benefits

Tips:

- Start with a smaller dose if new to castor oil
- Drink in the morning for optimal results

PEPPERMINT CASTOR TEA

Ingr:

- 1 tsp castor oil
- 1 tsp dried peppermint leaves
- 1 C. hot water
- 1 tsp honey

Proc:

- Steep dried peppermint leaves in hot water for 5 minutes
- Strain the tea and add castor oil and honey
- Stir well and drink warm

Benefits:

- Relieves digestive discomfort and bloating
- Soothes the digestive tract
- Refreshing and calming

Tips:

- Drink after meals for best results
- Adjust the amount of honey to taste

CASTOR OIL DETOX SMOOTHIE

Ingr:

- 1 Tbls castor oil
- 1 C. fresh pineapple chunks
- 1 C. spinach leaves
- 1 C. coconut water
- 1 small banana

Proc:

- Blend pineapple, spinach, coconut water, and banana until smooth
- Add castor oil and blend again until fully mixed
- Serve immediately

Benefits:

- Promotes detoxification and hydration
- Supports digestive health
- Provides essential vitamins and minerals

Tips:

- Use fresh ingredients for the best taste
- Drink as a breakfast smoothie for a healthy start to the day

CASTOR OIL HERBAL INFUSION

Ingr:

- 1 Tbls castor oil
- 1 tsp chamomile flowers
- 1 tsp fennel seeds
- 1 C. hot water

Proc:

- Steep chamomile flowers and fennel seeds in hot water for 10 minutes
- Strain the infusion and add castor oil
- Stir well and drink warm

Benefits:

- Calms the digestive system
- Reduces gas and bloating
- Promotes relaxation and stress relief

Tips:

- Drink before bedtime to aid digestion and promote sleep
- Can be sweetened with a bit of honey if desired

CASTOR OIL APPLE CIDER TONIC

Ingr:

- 1 Tbls castor oil
- 1 Tbls apple cider vinegar
- 1 C. warm water
- 1 tsp honey

Proc:

- Mix apple cider vinegar and honey in warm water
- Add castor oil and stir well until completely blended
- Drink on an empty stomach

Benefits:

- Boosts digestive health and metabolism
- Aids in detoxification
- Balances stomach acidity

Tips:

- Drink in the morning for best results
- Use raw, unfiltered apple cider vinegar for added benefits

DIGESTIVE CASTOR OIL PUDDING

Ingr:

- 1 Tbls castor oil
- 1 C. unsweetened almond milk
- 2 Tbls chia seeds
- 1 tsp vanilla extract
- 1 tsp honey

Proc:

- Combine almond milk, chia seeds, vanilla extract, and honey in a bowl
- Add castor oil and mix well
- Refrigerate for at least 4 hours or overnight

Benefits:

- Supports digestive health
- Provides a nutritious and filling snack
- Rich in fiber and omega3 fatty acids

Tips:

- Top with fresh fruits for added flavor
- Great as a healthy breakfast or dessert

CASTOR OIL CITRUS REFRESHER

Ingr:

- 1 Tbls castor oil
- 1 C. freshly squeezed orange juice
- 1 C. sparkling water
- 1 tsp fresh mint leaves, chopped

Proc:

- Mix freshly squeezed orange juice and sparkling water in a glass
- Add castor oil and stir well until fully blended
- Garnish with chopped mint leaves and serve

Benefits:

- Refreshes and revitalizes the digestive system
- Provides a boost of vitamin C
- Helps in detoxification

Tips:

- Serve chilled for a refreshing drink
- Can be adjusted with more or less sparkling water to taste

CASTOR OIL GREEN DETOX SOUP

Ingr:

- 1 Tbls castor oil
- 1 C. kale leaves, chopped
- 1 C. broccoli florets
- 1 C. vegetable broth
- 1 clove garlic, minced

Proc:

- In a pot, bring vegetable broth to a boil and add kale, broccoli, and garlic
- Cook until vegetables are tender
- Remove from heat and blend until smooth
- Add castor oil and stir well

Benefits:

- Detoxifies and nourishes the body
- Supports digestive health
- Packed with vitamins and minerals

Tips:

- Serve warm as a starter or main dish
- Add a pinch of salt and pepper to taste

CASTOR OIL LEMON GINGER SHOTS

Ingr:

- 1 Tbls castor oil
- 2 Tbls freshly squeezed lemon juice
- 1 tsp grated ginger
- 1 tsp honey

Proc:

- Combine lemon juice, grated ginger, and honey in a small glass
- Add castor oil and mix well
- Drink immediately

Benefits:

- Boosts digestion and metabolism
- Provides a quick energy boost
- Helps in detoxification

Tips:

- Take in the morning for a refreshing start
- Can be diluted with a bit of water if the taste is too strong

CASTOR OIL BERRY BLEND

Ingr:

- 1 Tbls castor oil
- 1 C. mixed berries (blueberries, strawberries, raspberries)
- 1 C. plain Greek yogurt
- 1 tsp honey

Proc:

- Blend mixed berries and Greek yogurt until smooth
- Add castor oil and honey and blend again until fully mixed
- Serve immediately

Benefits:

- Promotes digestive health
- Provides antioxidants and probiotics
- Supports overall gut health

Tips:

- Use fresh or frozen berries for best results
- Perfect as a snack or breakfast option

5.2 FORMULAS FOR PAIN AND INFLAMMATION

TURMERIC CASTOR OIL BALM

Ingr:

- 2 Tbls castor oil
- 1 tsp turmeric powder
- 1 tsp beeswax

Proc:

- Heat castor oil and beeswax in a double boiler until beeswax melts
- Remove from heat and stir in turmeric powder
- Pour into a container and let it cool and solidify

Benefits:

- Reduces inflammation and pain
- Enhances skin healing
- Provides a soothing effect

Tips:

- Apply to affected areas and massage gently
- Use as needed for pain relief

CASTOR OIL ARNICA GEL

Ingr:

- 2 Tbls castor oil
- 1 Tbls arnica gel
- 5 drops lavender essential oil

Proc:

- Mix castor oil, arnica gel, and lavender essential oil until well blended
- Store in a small jar
- Apply to sore muscles and joints

Benefits:

- Relieves muscle aches and pains
- Reduces bruising and inflammation
- Promotes relaxation

Tips:

- Use after physical activity for best results
- Keep in a cool, dry place

PEPPERMINT CASTOR OIL RUB

Ingr:

- 2 Tbls castor oil
- 5 drops peppermint essential oil
- 5 drops eucalyptus essential oil

Proc:

- Mix castor oil with peppermint and eucalyptus essential oils
- Store in a glass container
- Apply to affected areas and massage gently

Benefits:

- Provides cooling relief to sore muscles
- Reduces inflammation
- Soothes and relaxes the body

Tips:

- Apply before or after exercise for best results
- Can be used for headaches by massaging onto temples

CASTOR OIL AND CLOVE COMPRESS

Ingr:

- 2 Tbls castor oil
- 1 tsp clove oil
- Warm cloth

Proc:

- Mix castor oil and clove oil
- Soak a warm cloth in the mixture
- Apply the cloth to the affected area and leave for 20 minutes

Benefits:

- Alleviates joint pain and stiffness
- Provides deep tissue relief
- Increases blood circulation

Tips:

- Use for arthritis pain
- Reheat the cloth as needed for continuous warmth

CASTOR OIL AND ROSEMARY MASSAGE OIL

Ingr:

- 2 Tbls castor oil
- 1 Tbls rosemary essential oil
- 1 Tbls olive oil

Proc:

- Mix castor oil, rosemary essential oil, and olive oil until well combined
- Store in a dark glass bottle
- Use as a massage oil on sore areas

Benefits:

- Reduces muscle pain and tension
- Enhances circulation
- Provides a relaxing aroma

Tips:

- Ideal for a full body massage
- Warm the oil slightly before use for added comfort

CASTOR OIL GINGER WRAP

Ingr:

- 2 Tbls castor oil
- 1 tsp grated ginger
- Warm cloth

Proc:

- Mix castor oil with grated ginger
- Soak a warm cloth in the mixture
- Apply the cloth to the affected area and cover with a dry towel for 30 minutes

Benefits:

- Provides deep muscle relief
- Reduces inflammation
- Enhances blood flow

Tips:

- Use for chronic pain areas
- Reapply as needed for continued relief

<table><tr><td>CHAMOMILE CASTOR OIL LOTION</td></tr></table>

Ingr:

- 2 Tbls castor oil
- 1 Tbls chamomile essential oil
- 1 C. unscented lotion

Proc:

- Mix castor oil, chamomile essential oil, and unscented lotion until well combined
- Store in a pump bottle
- Apply to sore areas as needed

Benefits:

- Soothes skin and reduces pain
- Provides antiinflammatory benefits
- Moisturizes the skin

Tips:

- Perfect for daily use
- Keep in a cool, dry place

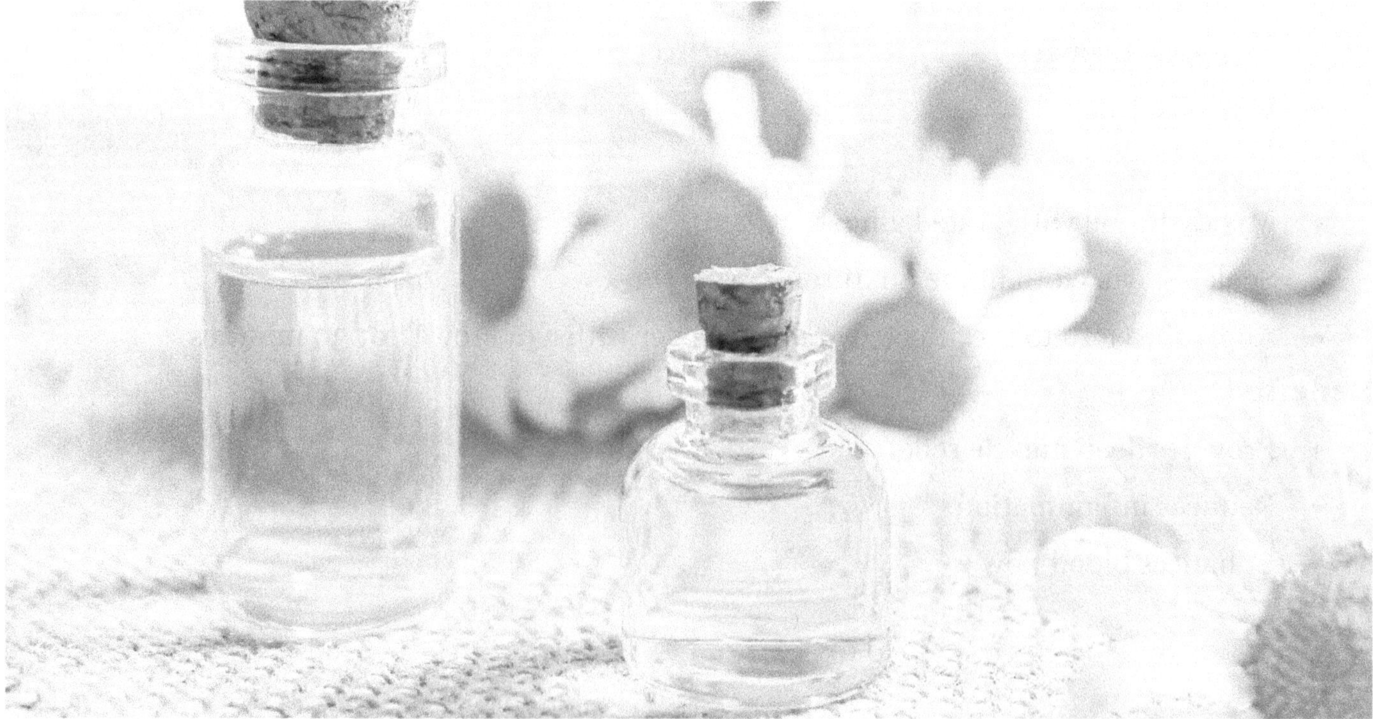

CASTOR OIL CAYENNE SALVE

Ingr:

- 2 Tbls castor oil
- 1 tsp cayenne pepper powder
- 1 tsp beeswax

Proc:

- Heat castor oil and beeswax in a double boiler until beeswax melts
- Stir in cayenne pepper powder until well mixed
- Pour into a container and let it cool and solidify

Benefits:

- Provides warming relief to sore muscles
- Reduces inflammation
- Stimulates blood flow

Tips:

- Apply to affected areas with caution to avoid sensitive skin
- Use sparingly to avoid irritation

LAVENDER CASTOR OIL BATH

Ingr:

- 2 Tbls castor oil
- 10 drops lavender essential oil
- Warm bath

Proc:

- Mix castor oil and lavender essential oil
- Add the mixture to a warm bath and stir well
- Soak in the bath for 2030 minutes

Benefits:

- Relaxes muscles and reduces pain
- Promotes overall relaxation
- Soothes the skin

Tips:

- Perfect before bedtime for a restful sleep
- Can be combined with Epsom salts for added benefits

CASTOR OIL WILLOW BARK BALM

Ingr:

- 2 Tbls castor oil
- 1 Tbls willow bark extract
- 1 tsp beeswax

Proc:

- Heat castor oil and beeswax in a double boiler until beeswax melts
- Remove from heat and stir in willow bark extract
- Pour into a container and let it cool and solidify

Benefits:

- Reduces pain and inflammation
- Provides a natural alternative to aspirin
- Soothes sore areas

Tips:

- Apply to affected areas as needed
- Keep in a cool, dry place for longlasting use

EUCALYPTUS CASTOR OIL CHEST RUB

Ingr:

- 2 Tbls castor oil
- 10 drops eucalyptus essential oil
- 5 drops lavender essential oil

Proc:

- Mix castor oil with eucalyptus and lavender essential oils until well combined
- Apply to the chest and throat area, massaging gently
- Cover with a warm cloth for enhanced absorption

Benefits:

- Clears nasal passages
- Relieves congestion
- Soothes the respiratory tract

Tips:

- Use before bedtime to promote better sleep
- Reapply as needed for continued relief

CASTOR OIL STEAM INHALATION

Ingr:

- 1 Tbls castor oil
- 1 liter hot water
- 5 drops tea tree essential oil

Proc:

- Add castor oil and tea tree essential oil to hot water in a large bowl
- Lean over the bowl, cover your head with a towel, and inhale the steam for 1015 minutes

Benefits:

- Clears sinuses
- Reduces symptoms of colds and sinusitis
- Provides antimicrobial benefits

Tips:

- Perform steam inhalation twice daily during respiratory issues
- Keep eyes closed to avoid irritation

PEPPERMINT CASTOR OIL VAPOR RUB

Ingr:

- 2 Tbls castor oil
- 10 drops peppermint essential oil
- 5 drops camphor essential oil

Proc:

- Mix castor oil with peppermint and camphor essential oils until well combined
- Apply to the chest, back, and throat, massaging gently
- Cover with a warm cloth for enhanced absorption

Benefits:

- Eases breathing
- Reduces coughing
- Soothes the respiratory tract

Tips:

- Use during colds and flu for best results
- Store in a cool, dry place

CASTOR OIL THYME INHALER

Ingr:

- 1 Tbls castor oil
- 10 drops thyme essential oil
- 1 small inhaler stick

Proc:

- Mix castor oil with thyme essential oil
- Pour the mixture into the inhaler stick
- Inhale deeply through the nose as needed

Benefits:

- Relieves respiratory congestion
- Provides antimicrobial benefits
- Supports overall respiratory health

Tips:

- Carry the inhaler with you for onthego relief
- Use at the first sign of respiratory discomfort

LAVENDER CASTOR OIL BREATHING BALM

Ingr:

- 2 Tbls castor oil
- 10 drops lavender essential oil
- 5 drops eucalyptus essential oil

Proc:

- Mix castor oil with lavender and eucalyptus essential oils until well combined
- Apply to the chest and under the nose, massaging gently
- Cover with a warm cloth for enhanced absorption

Benefits:

- Soothes the respiratory tract
- Promotes relaxation and restful sleep
- Reduces congestion

Tips:

- Use before bedtime for better sleep
- Reapply as needed for continued relief

CASTOR OIL GINGER RESPIRATORY TEA

Ingr:

- 1 Tbls castor oil
- 1 tsp grated ginger
- 1 C. hot water
- 1 tsp honey

Proc:

- Steep grated ginger in hot water for 5 minutes
- Strain the tea and add castor oil and honey, stirring well
- Drink warm

Benefits:

- Reduces throat irritation
- Soothes the respiratory tract
- Provides antiinflammatory benefits

Tips:

- Drink twice daily during respiratory issues
- Adjust ginger amount to taste

CASTOR OIL ROSEMARY STEAM BATH

Ingr:

- 1 Tbls castor oil
- 10 drops rosemary essential oil
- 1 liter hot water

Proc:

- Add castor oil and rosemary essential oil to hot water in a large bowl
- Lean over the bowl, cover your head with a towel, and inhale the steam for 1015 minutes

Benefits:

- Clears sinuses
- Reduces respiratory congestion
- Provides antibacterial benefits

Tips:

- Perform steam inhalation twice daily during respiratory issues
- Keep eyes closed to avoid irritation

CASTOR OIL LEMON EUCALYPTUS CHEST RUB

Ingr:

- 2 Tbls castor oil
- 10 drops lemon essential oil
- 10 drops eucalyptus essential oil

Proc:

- Mix castor oil with lemon and eucalyptus essential oils until well combined
- Apply to the chest and throat, massaging gently
- Cover with a warm cloth for enhanced absorption

Benefits:

- Relieves nasal congestion
- Eases breathing
- Soothes the respiratory tract

Tips:

- Use before bedtime for better sleep
- Reapply as needed for continued relief

CASTOR OIL BASIL INHALER

Ingr:

- 1 Tbls castor oil
- 10 drops basil essential oil
- 1 small inhaler stick

Proc:

- Mix castor oil with basil essential oil
- Pour the mixture into the inhaler stick
- Inhale deeply through the nose as needed

Benefits:

- Reduces respiratory congestion
- Provides antibacterial benefits
- Supports overall respiratory health

Tips:

- Carry the inhaler with you for onthego relief
- Use at the first sign of respiratory discomfort

CASTOR OIL SAGE STEAM INHALATION

Ingr:

- 1 Tbls castor oil
- 10 drops sage essential oil
- 1 liter hot water

Proc:

- Add castor oil and sage essential oil to hot water in a large bowl
- Lean over the bowl, cover your head with a towel, and inhale the steam for 1015 minutes

Benefits:

- Clears sinuses
- Reduces respiratory congestion
- Provides antimicrobial benefits

Tips:

- Perform steam inhalation twice daily during respiratory issues
- Keep eyes closed to avoid irritation

BOOK 2: "BEAUTY SECRETS OF CASTOR OIL: RADIANT SKIN AND LUSTROUS HAIR"

CHAPTER 1: CASTOR OIL FOR SKIN CARE

In the serenity of nature's own laboratory, a remarkable elixir for beauty—castor oil—has stood the test of time, weaving its way through history as a guardian of radiant skin and vital health. It is not by chance but by nature's design that castor oil, extracted from the humble seeds of the castor plant, emerges as a cornerstone in natural skincare. Its profound versatility can transform daily beauty practices, a testament celebrated in cultures around the globe.

Imagine a time when ancient healers found solace and power in the viscous, golden liquid, utilizing it to treat ailments and enhance natural beauty. Today, as we seek to return to more sustainable, gentle means of caring for our skin amidst the harsh chemicals prevalent in modern cosmetics, castor oil stands resolute—a beacon of simplicity and efficacy.

Castor oil's journey from seed to skin is a narrative of purity and vitality. This oil, dense with ricinoleic acid known for its antiinflammatory properties, acts not just on the surface but penetrates deeply, soothing, repairing, and hydrating the skin in ways synthetic products can scarcely manage. Whether it's integrating this golden oil into your daily moisturizing regimen or finding natural solutions to tackle acne, scars, or signs of aging, castor oil offers a pathway to not only enhanced beauty but also to a profound connection with the healing virtues of nature.

Take a moment to consider your own skincare routine: the array of bottles, the promises on their labels, the fleeting trends. Now picture this: a single bottle of castor oil, a natural aligning with life's simpler, more authentic paths. Through this chapter, we journey together through practical, actionable ways to redefine what it means to give your skin the utmost care and nourishment. Every application is a step closer to harnessing the allencompassing benefits of nature's own remedy, proving that sometimes, the most profound impacts come from the simplest sources.

1.1 DAILY SKIN CARE REGIMENS

Every morning welcomes a new opportunity to foster beauty that feels as good as it looks—a beauty that thrives on the purity and effectiveness of nature's gifts. Among these, castories oil, with its rich, healing attributes, plays a pivotal role in daily skin care. Its application is an ancient ritual, modernized by science to fit perfectly into the contemporary skincare mosaic.

Incorporating castor oil into your daily skin care regimen is akin to building a bridge back to nature.

Its unique, viscous consistency allows it to penetrate deep into the skin, providing nutrients and moisture that can rejuvenate and protect the epidermis from the environmental challenges we face daily. This daily application of castor oil facilitates not just a superficial vanity but a deeper, more sustainable form of selfcare that respects your body's natural rhythms and the environment.

Imagine the gentle, emboldening touch of the morning sun. Similarly, a morning routine using castor oil can invigorate and prepare your skin for the day ahead. Starting with a cleansed face, a light, massage with castor oil can stimulate blood circulation, enhancing the skin's natural healthy glow. This oil can be used as a standalone cleanser or a serum, depending on your skin's individual needs and responses. Not only does it clear the skin of impurities, but its fatty acids also offer potent moisturizing properties.

As the day winds down, your skin deserves a retreat—a moment to repair and breathe. Here, castor oil steps in once again as a powerful ally. At night, its use in your skincare routine can help to repair the wear and tear of daily life. Its compounds work to promote healing, reduce inflammation, and maintain the skin's moisture barrier throughout the night. This nightly application not only encourages the skin's process of regeneration but also relaxes the mind, thereby supporting an overall sense of wellbeing that can improve sleep quality.

Beyond its hydrating and healing properties, the protective function of castor oil cannot be understated. As a natural antibacterial agent, it safeguards the skin against environmental pollutants and pathogens that contribute to aging and disease. This protective layer ensures that your skin's defense system is supported and strengthened day after day.

Yet, the benefits of castor oil extend beyond individual use. Opting for castor oil as a staple in your skincare routine is also a choice for sustainability. In a world increasingly burdened by chemical pollutants and unsustainable practices, using castor oil—a biodegradable and easily produced natural product—lessens the ecological footprint of your beauty regimen. This aligns your personal care with a broader responsibility towards environmental stewardship, making each application an act of conscious living.

The transformative journey of incorporating castor oil into your daily skin care not only embellishes your skin but also entwines your personal health with the rhythms of the natural world. It is a testament to the simplicity and power of returning to nature for personal care solutions that not only ensure beauty but a profound equilibrium with the world around us.

Thus, embracing castor oil in daily skin care routines is more than a cosmetic practice; it is a holistic ritual that nurtures the skin, respects the environment, and enhances overall wellbeing. It underscores the philosophy that true beauty is rooted in health and sustainability, resonating with the body's natural processes and the planet that nourishes us.

The continued use of castor oil not only promises a transformation in how your skin feels and looks but also in how you relate to the world—beauty intertwined with health and consciousness. Through this daily commitment, you step into a lifestyle where beauty and wellness walk hand in hand, guided by the wisdom of nature and the powerful, nurturing essence of castor oil.

1.2 TREATMENT FOR ACNE AND BLEMISHES

In the world of skincare, few conditions seem as common yet as challenging as acne and skin blemishes. These pesky, often stubborn issues are bane of teenagers and adults alike, echoing concerns and frustrations across ages and cultures. However, nestled within the gentle, nurturing embrace of nature lies a formidable ally in castor oil. Renowned for its deep cleansing and antiinflammatory properties, castor oil offers those afflicted with acne a beacon of hope and healing.

Diving into the heart of acne treatment, castor oil stands out due to ricinoleic acid, a unique fatty acid that is highly effective in purifying and repairing the skin. This key component gives castor oil its distinctive ability to penetrate deep into the skin layers, dislodging debris and bacteria trapped under the skin's surface, thus preventing the eruptions that manifest as acne.

For anyone grappling with acne, the journey often begins with disillusionment—countless products promising miracles yet delivering little. In contrast, the approach with castor oil is grounded in simplicity and purity. Imagine starting your day by massaging your face with a few drops of this golden oil. This simple act can improve blood circulation, enhance lymphatic drainage, and facilitate the healing of inflamed skin. When integrated consistently into morning and evening routines, it methodically breaks down impurities, ensuring each new day progressively reveals clearer, smoother skin.

Beyond just treatment, castor oil sets the stage for prevention. Its antibacterial qualities tackle one of the root causes of acne—bacterial growth. By applying it to the skin, one establishes a barrier not just against existing bacteria, but also against external factors that contribute to recurrent acne flareups. Furthermore, for those whose skin scars easily from acne, castor oil may serve as a blessing. Its ability to promote collagen and elastin production not only reduces the appearance of scars but also enhances the skin's texture and elasticity.

While it's tempting to seek out drastic measures and harsh chemicals to deal with acne, castor oil invites us to embrace a gentler approach. This process of reintroducing more natural elements into our care regimen not only benefits our skin but also aligns our habits more closely with ecofriendly practices. Choosing castor oil over chemically laden treatments not only alleviates our skincare woes but also contributes to a healthier planet.

The calming routine of incorporating castor oil can transform what is often an anxietyfilled, reactive relationship with our skin into a proactive, nurturing ritual. It's a daily reaffirmation that gentle and steady care often leads to lasting results. Through this approach, individuals are not just combating acne but are also nurturing their skin with every application, promoting a healthier complexion that extends beyond mere appearance.

Moreover, in adopting castor oil as a cornerstone of acne treatment, there's an intrinsic lesson in patience and persistence—virtues necessary for any natural remedy. The beauty of this method lies not in instantaneous results but in the gradual, affirming shift towards balance and clarity in one's skin. Each day's application is a step forward in restoring the skin's natural harmony and vitality.

Thus, the narrative of treating acne and blemishes with castor oil is woven with threads of healing, sustainability, and holistic care. It encourages a deeper understanding and connection with our bodies, urging us to listen and respond with natural solutions that honor our health and the environment. In this light, castor oil is more than just a treatment; it's a testament to the power of returning to roots, utilizing Earth's offerings to heal and enhance our lives, proving that sometimes, the best solutions are the simplest, drawn straight from nature's own wisdom. Through castable oil, we find not only a remedy for acne but a path to living more harmoniously within our skin and our environment.

1.3 ANTIAGING AND WRINKLE REDUCTION

In the narrative of aging, where each line and wrinkle tells a story of laughter, worry, and the rich passage of time, many seek ways to soften these stories etched into their skin. Castor oil, a timeless elixir, offers itself as a gentle yet potent ally in the quest for ageless beauty. Unlike harsh chemical treatments that promise rapid results but often exacerbate skin frailty, castor oil works harmoniously with the body's natural processes to nurture and replenish aging skin, reducing wrinkles and enhancing skin resilience.

To understand the power of castor oil in antiaging and wrinkle reduction, one must delve into the science of skin itself. As we age, the production of essential proteins such as collagen and elastin—vital for skin's elasticity and firmness—diminishes. Environmental factors, lifestyle choices, and natural aging processes all contribute to the visible signs of aging. Here, castor oil's rich composition, loaded with fatty acids, antioxidants, and other bioactive compounds, plays a crucial role in fortifying the skin's integrity.

Castor oil's unique ability to penetrate deeply into the skin and nourish it from within makes it a remarkable natural remedy for aging skin.

It hydrates and lubricates the skin's layers, plumping out fine lines and making wrinkles less pronounced. Moreover, its antioxidant properties combat free radicals—molecules that accelerate aging and skin damage—thus protecting the skin's youthful appearance.

Imagine incorporating castor oil into your daily skin care routine as a ritual of selfcare that not only addresses aging concerns but also enhances overall skin health.

Each application is a moment of connection with the ageold wisdom of natural healing, providing a pause in our busy lives to nurture ourselves with the simplicity and purity of nature. This ritual not only feeds the skin but also nourishes the soul, reinforcing the connection between our physical exterior and internal health.

In the practice of using castor oil for antiaging, the methodology is as important as the product itself. Gentle massaging of the oil into the skin stimulates blood flow, which is crucial for regenerating new skin cells and maintaining skin vitality. This massage ritual transforms the routine from a mere skincare application into a therapeutic gesture of selflove and care, encouraging a meditative relationship with our aging selves.

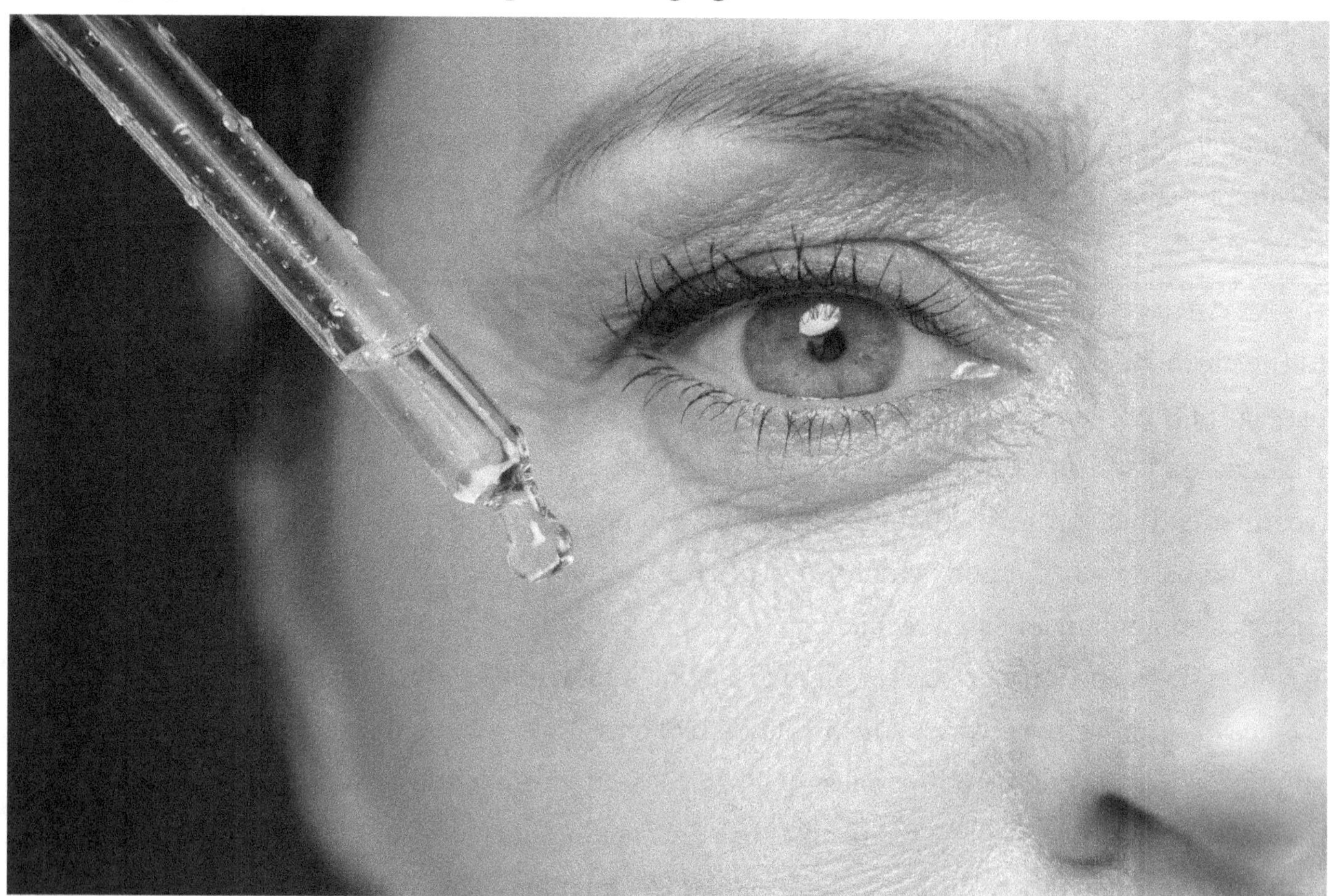

Beyond its direct application, castor oil's versatility extends into nighttime regimens where its intensive hydrating properties are especially beneficial. During sleep, our skin undergoes its most robust healing and regenerative processes.

Castor oil supports these natural cycles, its thick, nourishing texture forming a barrier that moisturizes and heals throughout the night, allowing you to awaken with a refreshed, more youthful appearance.

This approach to antiaging transcends the superficial goal of merely appearing younger; it's about embracing a holistic philosophy that appreciates aging as a natural and beautiful part of life's journey. Through consistent use of castor oil, one can maintain a vibrant, glowing complexion that reflects both personal health and the timeless beauty of nature itself.

Moreover, the choice of castor oil as a staple in your antiaging arsenal is also a gesture of environmental consciousness. In our modern world, where synthetic products and unsustainable practices abound, opting for a natural, easily renewable resource like castor oil minimizes our ecological footprint, aligning our beauty routines with a commitment to global stewardship.

Thus, in the realm of natural beauty, castor oil is not merely a substance but a symbol of the harmonious interaction between nature, health, and beauty. It invites us to redefine beauty standards, to embrace aging not as a battle but as an embrace, a celebration adorned with the wisdom of natural wellness. Whether smoothing over fine lines or deeply hydrating parched skin, castor oil remains a testament to the enduring power of natural remedies.

Through its use, we not only preserve our skin's youthfulness but also connect with the broader narrative of sustainable, conscious living—beauty care that cares for the world.

CHAPTER 2: NOURISHING HAIR TREATMENTS

Imagine the softness and sheen of wellnurtured hair gliding through your fingers. This dream can become your reality with the transformative powers of castor oil—a true elixir in the realm of hair care. As we embark on this chapter, I invite you to explore with me the miraculous ways castor oil can not only foster robust hair growth but also remedy the alltoocommon issues of dandruff and scalp health, paving the way to a crown full of healthy, vibrant hair.

Throughout my years delving into natural beauty solutions, the reverent tales of castor oil's efficacy from hundreds of individuals who have enhanced their hair's health are nothing short of inspiring. This golden, thick oil, extracted from the seeds of the Ricinus communis plant, stands as a pillar of strength in the natural beauty world. It serves not just as a product but as a timeless beauty tradition passed down through generations, each era discovering yet more innovative uses for it.

In this narrative, let us begin by understanding how the unique properties of castor oil, particularly its rich content of ricinoleic acid, imbue it with the ability to moisturize the scalp deeply, strengthening roots and preventing hair breakage. From here, I'll take you through personalized stories where individuals conquered the frustrating battle with dandruff, thanks to the antifungal properties of this oil.

And yet, the journey doesn't stop at nurturing the roots and scalp. Imagine a routine where the very act of massaging your hair with a mixture crafted from nature's finest, encourages not just physical growth but also a moment of calm and personal care in your busy life. The reflective gleam off of your hair after consistent treatment can mirror the serenity and health that castor oil promises.

As we proceed, you'll find tailored recipes that blend practicality with pampering—each designed to address different hair types and concerns. Whether your hair is perpetually dry, prone to frizziness, or lacks vitality, there's a castor oil solution waiting to breathe new life into every strand. Let's embark on this journey of transformation together, turning the pages toward a chapter of lush, thriving hair.

2.1 SOLUTIONS FOR HAIR GROWTH

In the pursuit of lush, voluminous hair, countless individuals have turned to a myriad of products, each promising the secret to rapid and robust hair growth. Yet, amidst this crowded landscape of temporary solutions and fleeting trends, castor oil emerges as a beacon of enduring efficacy. Renowned for its profound nourishing properties, this natural elixir offers more than mere conditioning—it stimulates the very foundation of healthy hair growth.

The journey to understanding how castor oil benefits hair begins at the root—quite literally. This oil's potency primarily comes from its rich concentration of ricinoleic acid, an essential fatty acid known to stimulate the scalp's blood circulation. Enhanced blood flow to the scalp ensures better nourishment for the hair follicles, which in turn fosters stronger, more resilient hair growth.

Moreover, castor oil's efficacy as a moisture sealant can combat the common yet troublesome issue of scalp dryness. A dry scalp can significantly hinder hair growth, leading to brittle, weak strands that are more susceptible to breakage. By maintaining adequate moisture, castor oil keeps the scalp environment optimally balanced, encouraging hair to not only grow but to thrive.

Personal stories lend credence to the theoretical benefits of castor oil. Take, for instance, Maria, a middleaged school teacher who once struggled with thinning hair. Despite trying various highend products, it was castor oil that finally made a noticeable difference. By integrating a weekly castor oil routine, Maria experienced a remarkable transformation, witnessing new hairs sprouting within just a few months, a sight she found both exhilarating and heartening.

Such anecdotal evidence is supported by the oil's rich nutrient profile. Aside from ricinoleic acid, castor oil is laden with omega6 and omega9 fatty acids, vitamin E, and other vital minerals—all of which are necessary for healthy hair texture and growth. This complex composition ensures not only the activation of hair growth but also increases the tensile strength of each hair strand, reducing the likelihood of split ends and hair breakage.

The benefits extend beyond the physical to the psychological. Incorporating castor oil into a hair care routine can become a therapeutic ritual. The simple act of massaging the oil into the scalp calms the mind, reducing stress levels which are often a contributing factor to hair loss. This holistic approach not only augments the health of the hair but also enriches the individual's overall wellbeing, creating a harmonious balance between mental and physical health.

Detractors might express concern about the oil's viscosity, fearing it might be too heavy or greasy for regular use. However, moderation and correct application techniques can mitigate these concerns, allowing individuals to reap the benefits without inconvenience. For example, diluting castic oil with lighter oils such as almond or coconut oil can enhance its spreadability and absorption, making the routine more enjoyable and less cumbersome.

While it's tempting to view castor oil as a miraculous cureall, it's essential to approach its use with a realistic perspective. Not every individual will experience the same results, nor will the changes occur overnight. Hair growth is a gradual process influenced by a variety of factors, including genetics, diet, and overall health. Therefore, patience and consistency become vital components in realizing the full benefits of castor oil.

In addition to its direct benefits on hair, castor oil also indirectly aids growth by preventing various scalp conditions. Its antibacterial and antifungal properties protect the scalp from infections that can cause hair follicle damage, ensuring that each follicle remains healthy and functional. This preemptive action not only secures the existing hair but also ensures a healthy environment for new growth.

Concluding with a broader perspective, castor oil's role in hair care exemplifies a larger movement toward natural and sustainable beauty practices. In an era where the impacts of synthetic chemicals are increasingly scrutinized, turning to natural solutions like castor oil not only benefits personal health but also contributes to a more environmentally conscious approach to beauty. This aligns with a collective shift towards products that offer safety, efficacy, and ethical production.

Embracing castor oil for hair growth is therefore not just a personal choice, but a lifestyle adjustment that echoes a global shift towards holistic wellbeing. Its comprehensive benefits illustrate not only the power of nature's offerings but also the importance of harnessing such pure resources responsibly and thoughtfully. As we continue to explore and understand the full spectrum of castor oil's capabilities, its integral role in natural beauty care remains clear and compelling, offering a timeless solution in the modern quest for health and vibrancy.

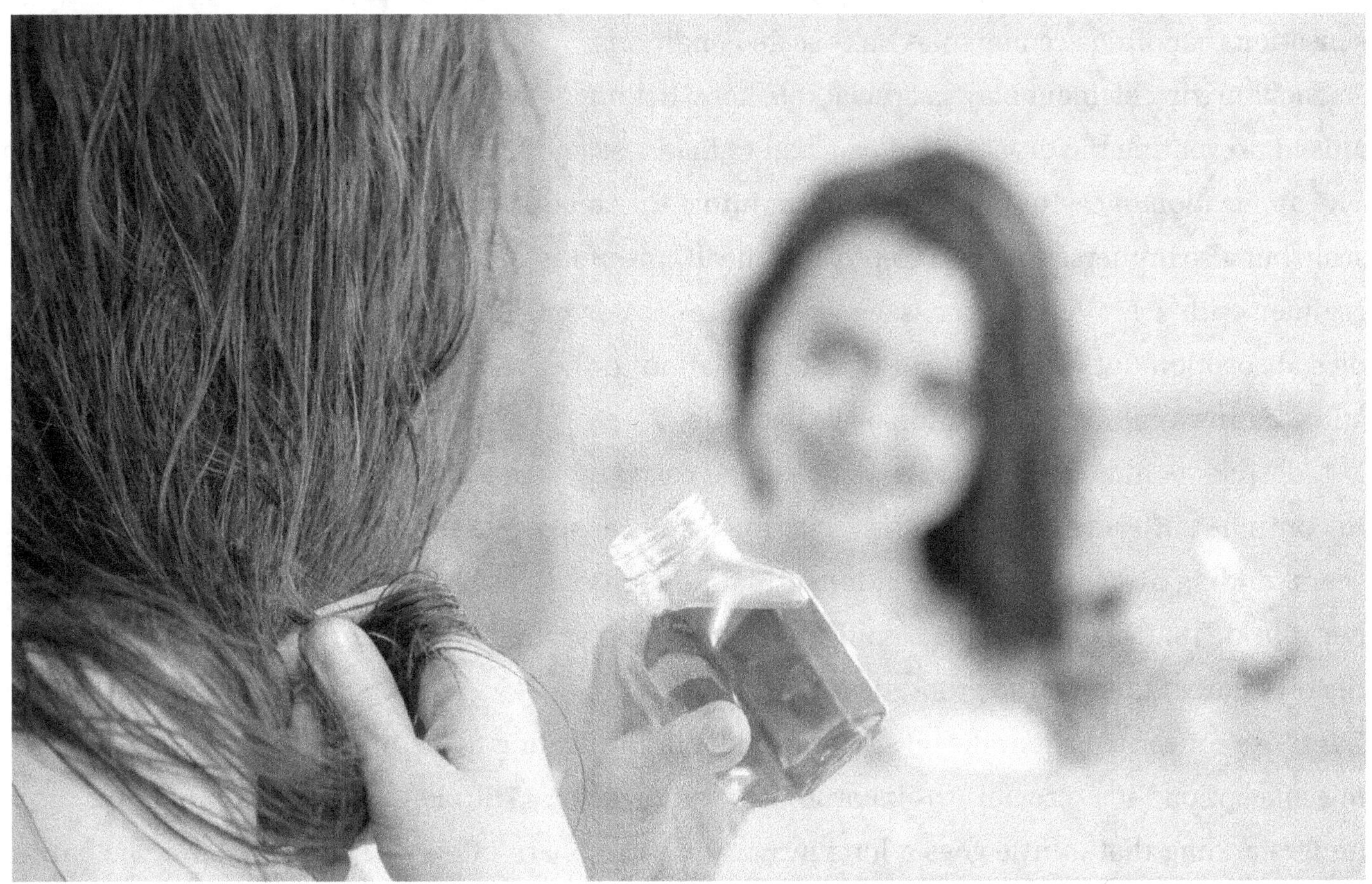

Dandruff and scalp issues—common yet often vexing problems that many face—can be both an aesthetic nuisance and a source of discomfort. Traditional approaches to treating such scalp conditions often involve harsh chemicals or shampoos that can strip the scalp of its natural oils. Here lies the remarkable efficacy of castor oil: an ageold remedy replete with healing properties that cater directly to the heart of scalp health issues without dogging the delicate balance of our scalp's ecosystem.

Understanding the causes of dandruff is fundamental to appreciating how castor oil functions as an effective remedy. Dandruff typically results from a dry scalp, but it can also be an outcome of excessive oil production that leads to seborrheic dermatitis. This condition is exacerbated by a yeast known as Malassezia, which thrives on the oils secreted by hair follicles. What makes castor oil so uniquely beneficial is its composition of ricinoleic acid, which not only combats fungal infections but also balances the scalp's pH level, creating an environment less favorable for dandruffcausing yeast to flourish.

But the benefits of castor oil extend beyond mere correction of fungal imbalance. It is also imbued with antiinflammatory properties that soothe irritated scalps, reducing redness and the itchy sensation that often accompanies flaky scalp conditions.

Its moisturizing element plays a crucial role here, helping to hydrate the scalp deeply. This in turn aids in preventing the dryness that can lead to flakiness and further scalp irritation.

The application of castor oil can transform into a therapeutic ritual that doesn't merely treat the scalp but also immerses one in a comforting, healthpromoting experience. Imagine beginning your regimen with a gentle scalp massage using warm castor oil. This method not only facilitates the oil's absorption but also enhances blood circulation to the scalp, promoting healthy hair growth and creating a calming moment in one's busy life.

Yet, despite its numerous benefits, the utility of castyl oil is not universally known, leading some to continue suffering in silence. Jasmine, for instance, struggled with seborrheic dermatitis for years, finding little relief in conventional treatments. It was only after integrating castor oil into her routine that she observed a significant reduction in scalp flakiness and itching—testament to the oil's potent therapeutic properties.

For those concerned about the oil's richness potentially leading to an overly oily scalp—a common misconception—it's crucial to incorporate it correctly. The key lies in moderation and understanding that a little goes a long jway. A few drops are often sufficient to cover the entire scalp area, thereby providing the healing benefits without the excess oiliness.

Moreover, integrating castor oil into one's hair care regime doesn't just respond to current problems but acts as a preventative measure, offering continuous nourishment that guards against the reappearance of scalp issues. In this sense, castor oil is more than a treatment; it's a sustainable practice, aligning with a broader shift towards natural and preventive health care.

The stories of those who've turned their scalp health around with castor oil also highlight an often overlooked aspect: the psychological impact of scalp issues. For many, persistent dandruff can erode confidence and increase social anxiety. Here, castor oil not only heals physically but restores a person's selfimage and mental wellbeing, underscoring the holistic impact of natural treatments. Further underscoring its efficacy, castor oil's antibacterial properties additionally protect the scalp from potential bacterial infections that can exacerbate or mimic the symptoms of dandruff, providing a comprehensive approach to scalp health that chemical treatments simply cannot match.

Reflecting a movement back to nature, the resurgence of interest in castor oil for dandruff and scalp health challenges the modern reliance on immediate, often superficial, chemical solutions. It invites us to reconsider traditional wisdom in the light of contemporary scientific validation, embracing a more empathetic and holistic approach to health care.

In sum, castor oil presents a profound yet simple solution to the complexities of scalp conditions. As it soothes, heals, and nourishes, this natural remedy reaffirms the connection between nature and human health, reminding us of our shared history with the natural world and inspiring a continued journey towards holistic wellbeing.

2.3 DEEP CONDITIONING AND SHINE ENHANCING

The quest for radiant, healthy hair that not only feels soft but also shines with a natural luster is often met with an array of products, each promising miraculous results. Amidst these, castor oil emerges as a profound agent for deep conditioning and enhancing the natural shine of hair. Its rich, nourishing properties penetrate deep into the hair shafts and lock in moisture, which is essential for correcting and preventing the brittleness and dullness often caused by environmental stressors and styling products.

Deep conditioning with castor oil is not just a remedy; it's an experience that transforms hair care into a ritual of renewal and nourishment. Its high concentration of fatty acids, particularly ricinoleic acid, makes it a powerful humectant, attracting and retaining moisture in the hair fibers. This capacity to deeply moisturize is pivotal not only for enhancing the hair's natural shine but also for fortifying each strand from the inside out, leading to a noticeable reduction in breakage and split ends.

The importance of maintaining a healthy moisture balance cannot be overstated. Hair that is wellmoisturized is less prone to tangling and snapping, which often results in hair loss and thinning. Here, castor oil's benefits extend beyond superficial aesthetics to improve hair health at its core. Moreover, this oil's ability to form a protective layer around the hair shaft helps shield the hair from harmful UV rays and environmental pollutants, factors that contribute to hair fading and keratin degradation over time.

In addition to its moisturization prowess, castor oil enhances the sheen of hair. A healthy, vibrant shine is the hallmark of hair that is in excellent condition. Castor oil facilitates this by smoothing the hair cuticles, which reflect light and produce a natural gloss. This smoothing effect is crucial, especially for those who regularly use heat styling tools that can roughen and damage the cuticle surface.

The process of applying castor oil for deep conditioning is both therapeutic and transformative. It begins with warming the oil slightly to thin it, making it easier to work through the hair and scalp. This warmth, combined with the rich texture of the oil, makes massaging it into the scalp a soothing experience—a moment of solace in the rush of daily life.

This massage not only facilitates deeper absorption but also stimulates blood flow to the scalp, promoting healthy hair growth and revitalization.

The universal appeal of castor oil lies in its simplicity and effectiveness. Regardless of hair type, texture, or condition, it offers a solution that is as beneficial for those with oily scalps as it is for those struggling with dryness. For instance, consider the story of Elena, who transformed her dry, lifeless hair into a cascading mane full of shine and vitality, all thanks to a consistent castor oil regimen. Such examples are numerous and speak volumes about the oil's versatile capabilities.

However, it's important to note that the results of castor oil treatment are cumulative. Consistency in application yields the best results, transforming hair gradually, restoring its health, and maintaining its beauty. The initial heaviness of the oil might dissuade some users, but its benefits far outweigh this minor inconvenience. Over time, users often find that their hair not only looks better but also feels stronger and healthier.

Castor oil is also cherished for its purity and sustainability. In a world increasingly inclined towards green beauty solutions, it stands out as a product that is both effective and environmentally friendly. It nourishes and beautifies without the need for synthetic additives or harmful chemicals, aligning with a more conscious approach to personal care.

Furthermore, the shineenhancing and conditioning properties of castor oil have communal implications.

They foster a shared beauty practice, uniting individuals across different generations and cultures in their pursuit of hair health. This shared experience enriches the practice, turning it into a legacy of beauty and health passed down through generations.

In conclusion, the role of castor oil in deep conditioning and enhancing shine is significant. It transcends mere cosmetic enhancement, touching the lives of its users by improving the health of their hair and, consequently, their selfconfidence. Whether it's through restoring moisture, protecting from damage, or simply adding a radiant sheen, castor oil continues to be an indispensable part of hair care routines worldwide, celebrated for its purity, effectiveness, and the profound connection it fosters with nature's healing properties.

CHAPTER 3: CASTOR OIL IN BEAUTY ROUTINES

In the transformative world of natural beauty, castor oil emerges not just as a mere ingredient but as a cornerstone in revolutionizing our daily beauty routines. As we delve into this chapter, you'll soon discover that integrating casting oil into your beauty rituals transcends conventional practice, invoking an art form that nurtures and restores natural radiance.

From the first tender swipe of castor oil across your eyelashes to the soothing application on your lips, each step in your beauty routine is an opportunity to connect with the timeless practices that have beautified generations. Readers often recount experiences of initial skepticism—how could something so simple transform their skin and hair? Yet, as they embraced castor oil, they noticed a definitive transformation, not just in their outward appearance, but in their overall sense of wellbeing.

Take, for instance, Mara, a dedicated nurse whose grueling hospital shifts left her little time for intricate beauty regimens. She integrated castor oil into her routine as a nightly moisturizer and lip salve. Gradually, her skin began to reveal its own story of resilience and renewal. Similarly, Tom, a father juggling career and home, found his rescue in castor oil for soothing postshave irritation and maintaining the lushness of his oftneglected hair. These stories underscore the simplicity and effectiveness of castor cave in your daily life offers a potent way to reconnect with the body's natural healing processes, while also ensuring each day begins with an act of selfcare.

As we proceed, you will learn how to seamlessly incorporate castford into routines that not only promise enhanced beauty but also an enriched spirit. Whether you're new to natural health products or a seasoned user of castor oil, the insights and recipes shared here aim to elevate your understanding and inspire a deeper commitment to a natural, radiant self. Thus, let us embark on this journey, exploring innovative uses and cherishing each drop of this golden elixir as we pave the way toward sustainable beauty practices.

3.1 INTEGRATING CASTOR OIL INTO MAKEUP REMOVAL

Throughout the years, I have met numerous individuals who have long sought a blend of beauty regimen that ticks all boxes; effective, natural, and soothing for the skin. Among the myriad of natural solutions I've explored, castor oil stands out as a hidden gem particularly effective in the delicate art of makeup removal.

The transition from makeupladen skin to its natural, refreshed state is more than just a nightly routine—it's a critical rejuvenation process for your skin.

Many don't realize that the typical makeup removers contain harsh chemicals that can strip natural oils from their skin, leaving it dry and irritated. Here, castor oil comes into play, offering not only to cleanse but also to replenish and heal.

Picture this: Ella, a professional makeup artist, was used to heavy, stubborn makeup both on herself and on her clients. The toll it took on her skin was evident, with premature fine lines and occasional breakouts. Her discovery of castor oil's benefits came as a revelation. She described how substituting her regular makeup remover with castor oil not only cleared away the makeup effectively but also improved the texture and health of her skin.

Why castor oil? Its high ricinoleic acid content, which is rare and highly effective in cleansing skin pores deeply while hydrating the skin. Furthermore, its natural antiinflammatory properties help in reducing redness and puffiness, often a result of frequent and prolonged makeup use.

Imagine another scenario involving Sam, a busy lawyer with minimal time for skincare routines. His introduction to castor oil was driven by his partner, a fervent advocate for natural living. Reluctant at first, Sam began using a simple mixture of castor oil for removing daily sunscreen and occasional makeup during social events. The easy application and the visible results in terms of smoother skin texture turned him into a believer.

Integrating castor oil into your makeup removal process isn't just about removing makeup but nurturing your skin's natural barrier. Its versatility extends to all skin types. Whether one has dry, oily, or sensitive skin, castor oil adjusts to meet individual skin needs, acting not just as a remover but as a skin conditioner.

Let's walk through how some have adapted castor oil into their lives for this purpose. Lina, for instance, a mother and an avid reader of natural health, mixes castor oil with a bit of almond oil to create a gentle yet effective makeup remover. This blend not only lifts away makeup but also ensures that her skin is infused with nutrients essential for repair and rejuvenation overnight.

Beyond the practicalities, incorporating castor oil into your evening ritual is an act of selfcare that goes deeper than the surface. It's about taking that moment to breathe, to gently massage and circulate this golden elixir onto your face, easing the stresses of the day away. This ritual not only cleanses the skin but also prepares your mind and body for a restful night's sleep, enhancing overall wellbeing.

However, transitioning to natural methods like using castor oil requires some adjustments. Initially, it might feel different or less effective than conventional removers because it doesn't contain aggressive stripping agents. But patience and consistency reveal its superiority, not only in maintaining the health of your skin but also in ensuring that you're nurturing your body in the most natural way possible.

The journey of integrating castor oil into standard beauty routines such as makeup removal is as much about embracing a holistic approach to skincare as it is about the practice itself. It champions a return to simplicity and purity in how we care for our skin—echoing a movement toward more sustainable and harmfree beauty practices.

For those who embark on this path, the transformation of their skin is just the beginning. They partake in a broader transformation—an awakening to the subtleties of natural wellness and beauty, grounded in the ageold wisdom that sometimes, the most profound benefits are found in the simplest of seeds. In this case, it's the humble yet mighty castor seed, a beacon of beauty, health, and renewal.

3.2 Hydrating Lips and Nail Care

The soothing touch of castor oil reaches beyond the surface, offering a balm not only for the skin but for the oftoverlooked parts of our body that work the hardest—our lips and nails. A blend of anecdotal wisdom and modern application has featured castor oil as an essential nurturing tool for these sensitive areas.

Let's delve into the narrative of Sofia, a pianist, whose evenings at the conservatory left her with painfully dry and chapped lips. Understandably, for someone who expresses herself through her music and gestures, maintaining comfortably hydrated lips is not merely cosmetic but essential. It was upon a friend's suggestion that she turned to caston oil. The thickness of the oil, she observed, provided a barrier against the elements while deeply hydrating the delicate skin of her lips. Sofia's experience is a testament to how small applications of such a natural, potent oil can result in significantly comforting outcomes.

Comparable to its effects on the lips, castor oil offers similar restorative properties to nail care. Consider the case of Alex, a craftsman whose daytoday life involves handling rough materials. The toll on his hands, and particularly his nails and cuticles, was an accepted part of his profession. However, the introduction to castor oil marked an unprecedented change. By merely rubbing a small amount of oil into his nails each night, he noticed not only an aesthetic improvement—his nails appeared shinier—but also a reduction in brittleness and peeling.

Moreover, the application of castor oil is not just a remedy but a preventive measure against common ailments affecting the nail bed and lip surface. Its antifungal and antibacterial properties serve as a protective shield, safeguarding against infections that can often complicate the health of one's nails and aggravate the condition of the lips.

For Claire, a stayathome mom, integrating castor oil into her family's daily routine was driven by her toddler's tendency to suffer from dry, cracked lips, especially in winter.

The safe, gentle nature of castor oil made it an excellent alternative to commercial products, which often contain chemicals or allergens that could irritate sensitive skin. Her relief at finding a solution that was both effective and healthconscious echoes a sentiment shared by many parents seeking safer health and beauty solutions for their families.

Transitioning to the broader topic of beauty and selfcare, the incorporation of castor oil into daily routines symbolizes a movement towards simpler, more grounded practices. It encourages an awareness of the ingredients in our products and their impact not only on our health but also on our environment. Using castor oil for lip and nail care is an act of nurturing that is both personal and environmentally considerate, minimizing exposure to synthetic substances and embracing a more sustainable approach.

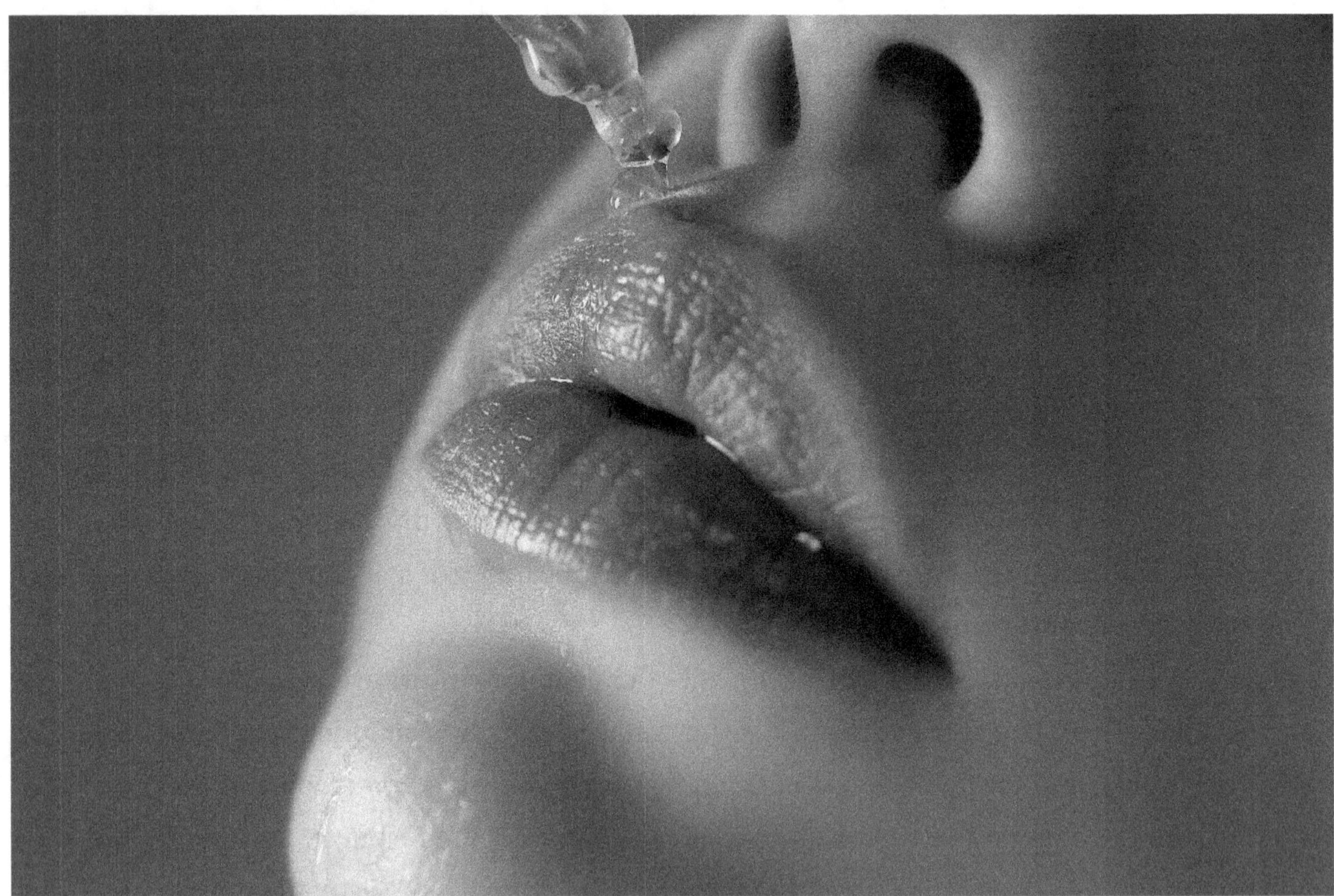

This shift towards natural remedies does not require grand gestures but can start with straightforward steps; a small bottle of castor oil and a few minutes can lay the foundation for a transformative selfcare ritual. In a world where the pace of life continues to accelerate, slowing down to care for oneself with natural, effective remedies offers a dual benefit: enhanced beauty and a reconnection with nature's rhythms.

The stories of those who have integrated castor oil into their beauty routines speak to the versatility and efficacy of this humble oil.

Each narrative reveals a layer of the holistic health portrait where castor oil is not only a supporting character but a star in its own right, spotlighting the oftenforgotten yet fundamental areas like our lips and nails.

Adopting such practices isn't just about treating dryness or combating brittleness; it's about investing in a process that honors the body's natural beauty and capacity for regeneration. Whether it's the protective application on a chilly day or the therapeutic ritual before bedtime, castor oil stands as a beacon of holistic care, inviting each of us to participate more fully in our health and to do so with grace and mindfulness.

Thus, the journey of incorporating castor oil into one's beauty regimen is as enriching as it is beautifying, reminding us that the most effective solutions are often the simplest and that the essence of beauty is, indeed, rooted in natural wellness.

3.3 ENHANCING EYELASHES AND EYEBROWS

In the realm of beauty where expressive eyes are celebrated, the desire for full, lustrous eyelashes and welldefined eyebrows has garnered a myriad of cosmetic solutions, ranging from serums to extensions. Yet, amidst these modern enhancements, castor oil emerges as a profoundly simple yet effective option to naturally accentuate the beauty of one's eyelashes and eyebrows.

This ageold remedy, cherished for its rich nutrients and natural growthstimulating properties, offers a gentle, sustainable alternative to the chemicalladen products that often populate the shelves.

Consider the experience of Julia, a graphic designer who found herself grappling with the effects of prolonged mascara use, which left her oncethick eyelashes sparse and brittle. The journey towards recovery began with skepticism but led to a surprising restoration, thanks to the consistent application of castor oil. Nightly, she would carefully apply a small amount of oil to her eyelashes with a clean mascara wand. Over time, not only did her lashes regain their original vigor and fullness, but they also exhibited a natural sheen that no mascara had ever achieved.

Similarly, the benefits of castor oil extend to managing and enhancing eyebrows. Michael, a seasoned actor, often altered his natural brows to fit various roles, which resulted in uneven growth and patches. Upon the recommendation of a makeup artist, who referred to castor oil as "nature's enhancer," Michael began applying a few drops to his eyebrows each evening. The transformation was gradual but undeniable, as the patches started to fill in, giving him more naturallooking, fuller brows without the need for frequent touchups with a pencil or gel.

The science behind castor oil's efficacy lies in its unique composition.

Rich in ricinoleic acid—a type of fatty acid with antiinflammatory properties—castor oil enhances blood circulation to the follicles, promoting healthier hair growth. Additionally, its moisturizing properties help to prevent hair breakage and nourish the hair at the roots, essential factors in achieving denser and more resilient lashes and brows.

For Anne, a teacher and mother of two, simplifying her beauty routine was not just a preference but a necessity given her busy lifestyle. She discovered that castor oil was not only beneficial for her eyelashes and eyebrows but was a multitasking product that she could use across her entire beauty regimen. Her story, shared often at community workshops, highlights the ease with which castor oil can be integrated into one's daily routine, proving that effective beauty solutions do not have to be complex or timeconsuming.

Beyond individual testimonies, the trend of using castor oil for eyelashes and eyebrows reflects a broader shift towards more holistic beauty practices. Consumers increasingly favor products that support longterm health and sustainability, both for themselves and the environment. In this context, castor oil is more than just a beauty product; it is part of a lifestyle choice that prioritizes wellness and natural living.

To those new to using castor oil, the approach is simple: start with a clean, spoolshaped brush for the eyelashes and a few drops of oil.

For eyebrows, a small brush or fingertip can be used to apply the oil directly along the brow line. Consistency is the key to seeing results; therefore, integrating this practice into the nightly routine enhances the likelihood of achieving the desired outcomes.

The collective experiences of those who have turned to castor oil reveal a pattern of positive outcomes not just in beauty enhancement but in fostering a deeper connection with natural wellness practices. Each story underscores a return to simplicity and purity in beauty routines, illustrating that sometimes the most effective solutions are gleaned not from the latest technological advancements but from the treasures found in nature.

In conclusion, incorporating castor the beauty routines of individuals around the world continues to reaffirm its effectiveness. With each application, users are not only enhancing their outward appearance but are also participating in an ageold tradition of natural selfcare—celebrating beauty in its most pure and sustainable form.

CHAPTER 4: SPECIALIZED BEAUTY APPLICATIONS

As we dive deeper into the exquisite world of castor oil and its virtually unlimited potential in beauty treatments, we now explore its specialist applications—a realm where the transformative powers of this golden elixir really shine. Beyond the daily grind of skin and hair care, castor oil emerges as a vital ally in addressing specific, often stubborn beauty concerns that range from dry, flaky skin to the more elusive perfect pedicure.

Imagine a world where your most troubling skin conditions, such as eczema or psoriasis, no longer dictate your choice of wardrobe or outings. Castor oil, with its potent antiinflammatory and hydrating properties, offers not just relief but a promise of healthier skin. Through the voices of countless individuals I have consulted, there echoes a common narrative of transformation and newfound confidence. It's not merely about treating symptoms but nurturing the skin to reveal its inherent vitality.

Our journey with castor oil also takes us to the oftenneglected extremities—our hands and feet. Here, the magic of this oil manifests in its ability to soften cuticles, heal cracked heels, and enhance the resilience of our nails. Each application is a step toward not only aesthetic enhancement but also functional health, facilitating our daily tasks and interactions.

In the cozy warmth of your home, castor oil can be your secret to a spalike pedicure or a soothing hand treatment. Picture a quiet evening, perhaps with soft music in the background, as you indulge in a castor oil soak. It's these moments of personal care that reinforce our connection with nature's remedies, turning routine into ritual.

This chapter is not just about occasional treatments. It's about integrating these rich, nourishing experiences into your life, crafting a beauty regimen that feels as luxurious as it is beneficial. I invite you to explore how castor oil can be more than just a product; it can be a catalyst for change, empowering you to take control of your beauty and health in the most natural way possible.

4.1 TREATMENTS FOR SKIN CONDITIONS (ECZEMA, PSORIASIS)

Navigating the complexities of skin conditions like eczema and psoriasis can be a profoundly personal, often challenging journey. These issues aren't just skin deep; they affect an individual's comfort, confidence, and even their social interactions. Amidst the vast landscape of treatments and advice, castor oil emerges as a soothing balm, rooted in the wisdom of nature, offering both relief and rejuvenation for troubled skin.

Eczema and psoriasis are primarily inflammatory conditions. They do not merely disturb the surface of your skin; they mirror disruptions from within—be it immune response, stress, or genetic factors. Traditional approaches often emphasize symptom management.

However, castor oil's approach is holistic, aiming to address both the symptoms on the skin's surface and the underlying inflammation.

The efficacy of castor oil in dealing with these skin conditions lies in its unique chemical composition. Ricinoleic acid, a rare constituent found abundantly in castor oil, is a powerful antiinflammatory agent. It works by penetrating the skin, easing inflammation, and hydrating the skin by retaining moisture, which is particularly beneficial for the dry and often flaky patches characteristic of eczema and psoriasis.

Moreover, the restoration of skin's moisture barrier is critical in managing these conditions, as compromised barrier can lead to more severe flareups. The moisturizing properties of castor oil not only soothe the skin but also protect it by helping to restore its barrier function. This dual action not only alleviates current discomfort but also aids in reducing the frequency and intensity of flareups.

In the context of natural remedies, the simplicity of castor oil is its strength. Its application can be integrated seamlessly into daily routines, providing a respite from the often harsh and irritating effects of some pharmaceutical treatments. For many, turning to a bottle of castor oil is not just a means of treating symptoms but is emblematic of adopting a gentler approach to personal health care—one that respects both the body and nature.

4.2 CASTOR OIL FOR FOOT AND HAND CARE

In the realm of beauty and personal care, the hands and feet often carry the burden of our daily endeavors yet seldom receive the pampering they deserve. From the artist who sculpts without rest, to the gardly who tends her garden, our hands and feet are essential tools that interact with the world in both bold and delicate ways. Castor oil, a gift from the castor plant, provides a deeply nourishing solution, not just soothing the wear and tear of daily life, but enhancing the resilience and beauty of these vital parts of our body.

Though it may seem simple, the care for hands and feet with castor oil is backed by a profound understanding of dermatology. Rich in ricinoleic acid, which has noteworthy antiinflammatory properties, and laden with moistureretaining triglycerides, castor oil offers an unrivaled treatment for dry, cracked skin which is common on hands and feet. These attributes make it an excellent choice for nurturing skin that is not only regularly exposed to the elements but also subject to frequent washing and potentially harsh chemicals.

Consider the commonplace challenge of dry heels, a condition that affects many and can lead to discomfort and even pain.

Regular application of castor oil can transform cracked heels, softening the skin and infusing it with moisture. This not only alleviates discomfort but also prevents further damage by maintaining the elasticity and resilience of the skin.

Similarly, for the hands, which are so often our interface with the world, castor oil provides more than just superficial beauty benefits. Its application strengthens the nails, softens cuticles, and enhances the skin's ability to guard against bacterial and fungal infections. Moreover, for those who experience eczema on their hands—a common but troubling problem—castor oil can be especially beneficial. Its antiinflammatory properties help to manage flareups, reducing redness and itching, and its emollient qualities help prevent new patches of dry, irritated skin from forming.

The application of castor oil to hand and foot care is both a science and an art. As a holistic remedy, it does not isolate the treatment of symptoms but supports the overall health of the skin. For example, in colder months, when the skin is particularly prone to becoming dry and brittle, the protective barrier that castor oil can offer is invaluable. It acts not just as a shield, guarding against harsh environmental factors, but also as a healer, restoring smoothness and elasticity.

For those who might initially turn to more complicated regimens and expensive products to care for their hands and feet, casty oil presents a beautifully simplistic yet profoundly effective alternative. Integrating this natural oil into daily routines does not require convoluted methods; often, it's as simple as massaging a small amount into the skin or nails regularly.

Beyond its practical applications, using castor oil is also a ritualistic act, encouraging slow, deliberate care that stands in contrast to the often hurried routines of modern life. It is an invitation to pause and engage with the body in a nurturing, intimate way. Whether it's a few moments spent massaging oil into tired feet at the end of the day, or caring for one's hands after a long day of work, these acts of care are grounding and meditative.

In the broader context of natural and sustainable beauty practices, castor oil is exemplary. It aligns with a mindful approach to personal care, where every ingredient is considered for both its efficacy and its impact on the world around us. In this light, choosing castor oil is not only a personal health decision but an ethical one, promoting a cycle of wellness that supports both the individual and the environment.

Utilizing castor oil for the care of hands and feet is not merely about addressing dryness or enhancing beauty. It is about reclaiming a tradition of holistic health, recognizing the hands and feet as deserving of as much care as the rest of our body. It's about embracing simplicity in a complex world and finding wellness in every drop of oil.

Thus, as we apply castor oil, we do more than treat our skin; we honor our bodies and acknowledge their hard work, promoting not just physical health but a profound, holistic wellbeing.

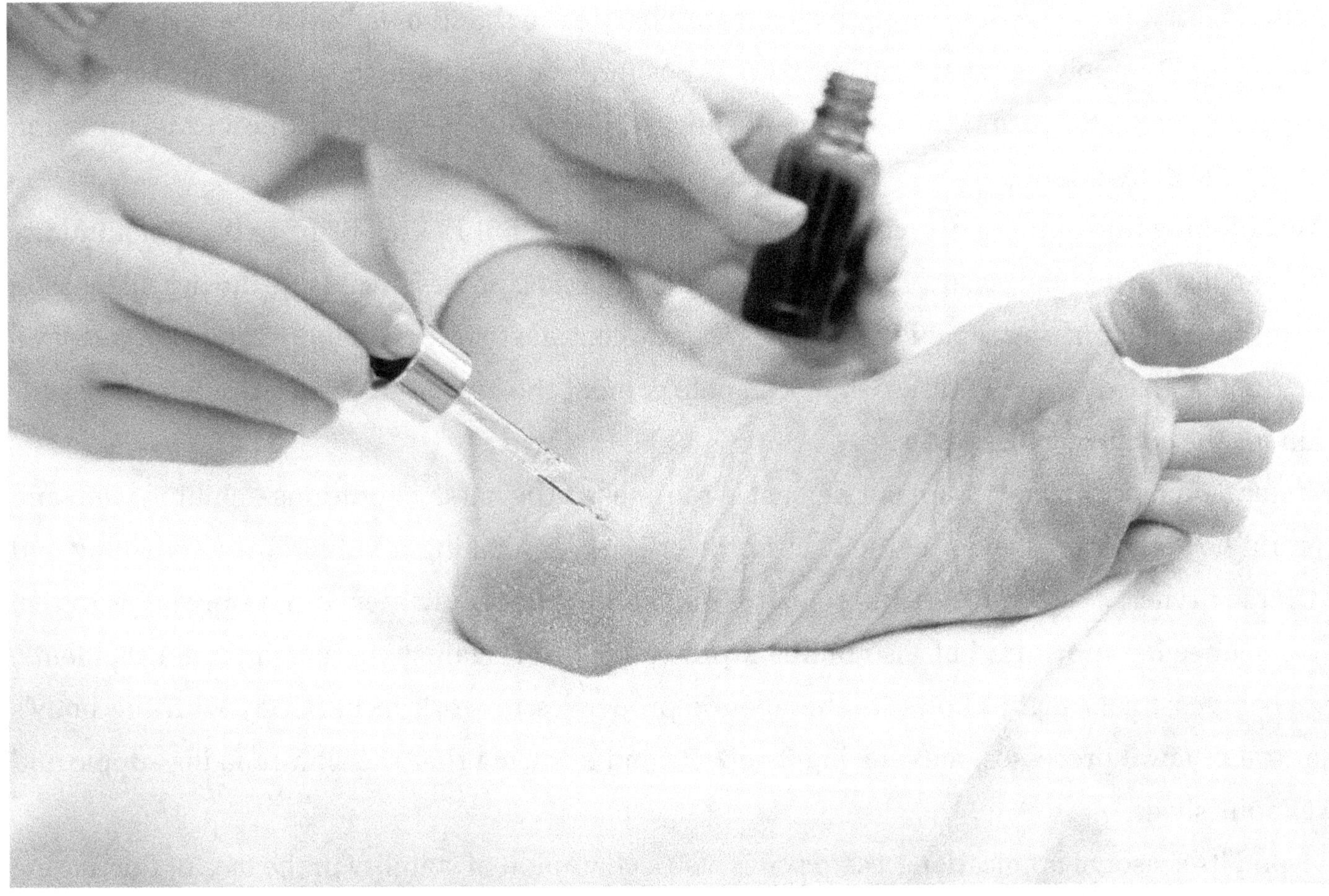

4.3 SEASONAL SKIN CARE TIPS WITH CASTOR OIL

Our skin is not just the barrier shield against the outer world, it also reflects the changing rhythms of the seasons. With each transition—from the blossoming warmth of spring to the crisp spells of autumn—our skin adjusts and reacts, sometimes struggling to maintain its natural balance. Understanding the seasonal needs of our skin can transform our approach to beauty routines, and in this delicate dance of change, castos oil plays a pivotal role in nurturing and protecting our skin throughout the year.

In the bloom of spring, as we shed the layers of clothing and embrace the mild warmth, our skin often emerges from the cold, dry months of winter feeling parched and sensitive. Spring is a time for rejuvenation, and castor oil can be particularly beneficial during this season for its ability to restore moisture and enhance elasticity. Its thick, emollient properties fill the cracks of winter dryness, preparing the skin to face the new season's elements with renewed strength.

As we move into summer, the vibrant sun beckons us outdoors, but not without its challenges for our skin.

High temperatures and increased exposure to ultraviolet light can lead to sunburns, and prolonged air conditioning can strip moisture from the skin. Here, castor oil's role shifts slightly. Its natural inflammatory properties and its ability to create a barrier on the skin make it an excellent aftersun treatment. By applying castor oil postsun exposure, you facilitate the skin's natural healing processes, soothing burns and reducing peeling, while simultaneously locking in moisture and preventing dehydration.

Transitioning into autumn, the crisp air can feel refreshing, but it often brings a drop in humidity that can lead to dry, flaky skin. Castor oil, with its fatty acids, proves invaluable during this season for its deep moisturizing capabilities. This is the perfect time to integrate more intensive castor oil treatments, like overnight masks which can help combat the increased dryness and prepare your skin for the coming cold months.

Winter demands the most from our defensive routines as the harsh conditions—chilling wind and central heating—can strip away the skin's protective layer, making it vulnerable to cracking and extreme dryness. Castor oil's rich, protective quality is critical in winter. It not only helps to seal in muchneeded moisture but also builds a protective layer against the harsh winter elements. Applying castor at night allows its therapeutic properties to work in harmony with the body's natural renewal processes, maximizing its effects and ensuring that the skin remains supple and wellnourished.

Beyond its seasonal applications, castor oil is also a champion of stability in the face of fluctuating environments. Its versatility makes it an ideal yearround companion, adapting to the specific needs of your skin in different climates and seasons. One of the most beautiful aspects of using castor oil in your skincare regimen is the way it encourages you to be attentive and responsive to the needs of your skin, promoting a kind of dialogue between you and your body.

This responsive approach is not just about combating the challenges of each season but also embracing the unique opportunities they bring. Spring offers the chance to revitalize, summer to protect, autumn to nourish deeply, and winter to fortify. Castor oil is an aid that supports throughout these cycles, fostering resilience in the skin's own natural defenses.

Adopting castor oil into your seasonal skincare routine speaks to a broader philosophy of wellness, where we heed the changing needs of our bodies and align our practices harmoniously with nature's cycles. This ongoing adjustment and tuning in is not just about maintaining appearance but about deep, sustained health that radiates from the inside out.

Thus, as each season changes, let castor oil guide you in nurturing not just your skin but your connection to the natural world. It is a humble, yet powerful reminder of how our care routines can mirror the ecological wisdom around us, teaching us to adapt, renew, and protect. As we follow the cycles of nature, we learn to care for ourselves with the same rhythm and respect, using castos oil as our companion in a lifelong journey of natural beauty and wellness.

CHAPTER 5: DIY BEAUTY RECIPES WITH CASTOR OIL

In the serene sanctuary of your home, you hold the power to transform your beauty routine into a nurturing ritual that celebrates nature's generosity. Castor oil, a humble yet miraculous elixir, has been revered for generations not just for its vast therapeutic qualities, but also as a cornerstone in beauty treatments that promise radiance and vitality. This chapter is your gateway to rediscovering beauty practices that align with the rhythms of the natural world, enticing you to explore concoctions within the quiet ambiance of your kitchen.

Imagine starting your day with a nourishing hair mask, whisked together with just a few spoons of castor oil combined with honey and perhaps a splash of coconut milk. This isn't merely a routine; it's a rebirth for your hair, offering deep conditioning and a sheen that mimics the golden sunlight. Transition to the evening, when your skin craves rest and rejuvenation. Here, castor oil blends seamlessly with essential oils, creating an enchanting potion that doesn't just cleanse but transforms your nighttime ritual into an act of selflove and care.

Each recipe provided in this chapter comes from a deep understanding of nature's profound impact on our wellbeing. As you leaf through these pages, you'll find more than just mixtures and methods; you'll discover stories of those who have woven these ingredients into their daily lives, finding solace in their soothing textures and scents. From a young mother who regained her confidence through a postpartum hair treatment to an elder who found solace in the gentle touch of a castor oilbased balm on weathered skin, these narratives thread together a tapestry of ageold wisdom and modernday testimonies.

As you embark on crafting your DIY beauty recipes, remember that each drop of castressor oil carries a beat of nature's heart. With every application, you are not only enhancing your outer beauty but are also embracing a tradition that honors the purity and power of the natural world. Let this journey be one of transformation, as you reinvent your beauty rituals to be as wholesome and enriching as the ingredients they contain.

CASTOR OIL ROSEHIP FACIAL SERUM

Ingr:

- 1 Tbls castor oil
- 1 Tbls rosehip oil
- 5 drops frankincense essential oil

Proc:

- Combine castor oil, rosehip oil, and frankincense essential oil in a small dropper bottle
- Shake well to mix
- Apply a few drops to clean skin and massage gently in upward motions

Benefits:

- Hydrates and nourishes the skin
- Reduces the appearance of fine lines and wrinkles
- Promotes a youthful glow

Tips:

- Use nightly before bed for best results
- Store in a cool, dark place to preserve potency

LAVENDER CASTOR OIL NIGHT CREAM

Ingr:

- 2 Tbls castor oil
- 1 Tbls shea butter
- 10 drops lavender essential oil

Proc:

- Melt shea butter in a double boiler until smooth
- Remove from heat and stir in castor oil and lavender essential oil
- Pour into a jar and let it cool to solidify

Benefits:

- Deeply moisturizes and repairs the skin overnight
- Soothes and calms irritated skin
- Promotes relaxation for better sleep

Tips:

- Apply to face and neck before bedtime
- Keep the jar tightly sealed to maintain freshness

ALOE VERA CASTOR OIL MOISTURIZER

Ingr:

- 1 Tbls castor oil
- 2 Tbls aloe vera gel
- 5 drops tea tree essential oil

Proc:

- Mix castor oil, aloe vera gel, and tea tree essential oil in a small bowl until well combined
- Apply to clean skin and massage gently until absorbed

Benefits:

- Hydrates and soothes the skin
- Helps clear acne and blemishes
- Provides a cooling sensation

Tips:

- Use morning and night for best results
- Store in the refrigerator for a refreshing application

BRIGHTENING TURMERIC CASTOR OIL MASK

Ingr:

- 1 Tbls castor oil
- 1 tsp turmeric powder
- 1 Tbls plain yogurt

Proc:

- Mix castor oil, turmeric powder, and plain yogurt in a bowl until well blended
- Apply an even layer to the face and leave on for 1520 minutes
- Rinse off with warm water

Benefits:

- Brightens and evens out skin tone
- Reduces dark spots and hyperpigmentation
- Provides a natural glow

Tips:

- Use once a week for best results
- Be careful with turmeric as it can stain clothing

EXFOLIATING CASTOR OIL SUGAR SCRUB

Ingr:

- 2 Tbls castor oil
- 1 C. granulated sugar
- 1 Tbls honey

Proc:

- Mix castor oil, granulated sugar, and honey in a bowl until well combined
- Gently massage onto damp skin in circular motions
- Rinse off with warm water and pat dry

Benefits:

- Exfoliates dead skin cells
- Leaves skin smooth and soft
- Enhances blood circulation

Tips:

- Use once or twice a week
- Store in an airtight container to prevent sugar from clumping

SOOTHING CHAMOMILE CASTOR OIL TONER

Ingr:

- 1 Tbls castor oil
- 1 C. chamomile tea (cooled)
- 1 tsp witch hazel

Proc:

- Brew chamomile tea and let it cool completely
- Mix castor oil, chamomile tea, and witch hazel in a small spray bottle
- Shake well before each use
- Spray onto clean skin and let it air dry

Benefits:

- Soothes and calms irritated skin
- Reduces redness and inflammation
- Refreshes and hydrates

Tips:

- Use daily after cleansing
- Store in the refrigerator for a cooling effect

ANTIAGING CASTOR OIL EYE CREAM

Ingr:

- 1 Tbls castor oil
- 1 tsp vitamin E oil
- 5 drops rose essential oil

Proc:

- Combine castor oil, vitamin E oil, and rose essential oil in a small jar
- Mix well until fully blended
- Gently apply a small amount around the eye area, tapping lightly with your fingertips

Benefits:

- Reduces fine lines and wrinkles around the eyes
- Hydrates and firms the delicate skin
- Diminishes dark circles

Tips:

- Use nightly before bed
- Be gentle when applying to avoid pulling the skin

HYDRATING CASTOR OIL LIP BALM

Ingr:

- 1 Tbls castor oil
- 1 tsp coconut oil
- 1 tsp beeswax

Proc:

- Melt beeswax and coconut oil in a double boiler until smooth
- Remove from heat and stir in castor oil
- Pour into small lip balm containers and let it cool to solidify

Benefits:

- Moisturizes and protects the lips
- Heals chapped and dry lips
- Provides a natural shine

Tips:

- Apply as needed throughout the day
- Keep in a cool, dry place to maintain consistency

REJUVENATING CASTOR OIL FACE MIST

Ingr:

- 1 Tbls castor oil
- 1 C. rose water
- 5 drops geranium essential oil

Proc:

- Mix castor oil, rose water, and geranium essential oil in a spray bottle
- Shake well before each use
- Spray onto face and neck as needed for a refreshing boost

Benefits:

- Hydrates and rejuvenates the skin
- Provides a natural glow
- Refreshes the skin throughout the day

Tips:

- Use anytime for a quick pickmeup
- Store in the refrigerator for an extra cooling effect

CLARIFYING CASTOR OIL CLAY MASK

Ingr:

- 1 Tbls castor oil
- 1 Tbls bentonite clay
- 1 Tbls apple cider vinegar

Proc:

- Mix castor oil, bentonite clay, and apple cider vinegar in a bowl until smooth and pastelike
- Apply an even layer to the face and leave on for 1015 minutes
- Rinse off with warm water and pat dry

Benefits:

- Detoxifies and purifies the skin
- Clears pores and reduces acne
- Leaves skin feeling fresh and clean

Tips:

- Use once a week for best results
- Avoid using metal utensils when mixing the clay

CASTOR OIL HAIR GROWTH SERUM

Ingr:

- 2 Tbls castor oil
- 1 Tbls jojoba oil
- 10 drops rosemary essential oil

Proc:

- Mix castor oil, jojoba oil, and rosemary essential oil in a small dropper bottle
- Shake well to combine
- Apply a few drops to the scalp and massage gently in circular motions

Benefits:

- Stimulates hair growth
- Strengthens hair roots
- Improves scalp health

Tips:

- Use 23 times a week for best results
- Store in a cool, dark place to preserve potency

HYDRATING CASTOR OIL HAIR MASK

Ingr:

- 2 Tbls castor oil
- 1 ripe avocado, mashed
- 1 Tbls honey

Proc:

- Combine castor oil, mashed avocado, and honey in a bowl
- Mix until smooth and well blended
- Apply to damp hair from roots to ends and leave on for 30 minutes
- Rinse thoroughly with warm water

Benefits:

- Deeply moisturizes and nourishes hair
- Adds shine and softness
- Repairs damaged hair

Tips:

- Use once a week for optimal hydration
- Cover hair with a shower cap to avoid dripping

COCONUT CASTOR OIL CONDITIONER

Ingr:

- 2 Tbls castor oil
- 2 Tbls coconut oil
- 1 tsp vitamin E oil

Proc:

- Mix castor oil, coconut oil, and vitamin E oil until well combined
- Apply to damp hair after shampooing
- Leave on for 510 minutes
- Rinse thoroughly with warm water

Benefits:

- Conditions and detangles hair
- Adds shine and softness
- Strengthens hair strands

Tips:

- Use every wash for best results
- Store in a cool, dry place to maintain consistency

CASTOR OIL AND ALOE VERA SCALP SOOTHER

Ingr:

- 2 Tbls castor oil
- 2 Tbls aloe vera gel
- 5 drops tea tree essential oil

Proc:

- Combine castor oil, aloe vera gel, and tea tree essential oil in a bowl
- Mix well until smooth
- Apply to the scalp and massage gently
- Leave on for 1520 minutes
- Rinse thoroughly

Benefits:

- Soothes itchy and irritated scalp
- Reduces dandruff
- Promotes a healthy scalp

Tips:

- Use twice a week for relief
- Store in the refrigerator for a cooling effect

LEMON CASTOR OIL CLARIFYING RINSE

Ingr:

- 1 Tbls castor oil
- 2 Tbls lemon juice
- 1 C. distilled water

Proc:

- Mix castor oil, lemon juice, and distilled water in a spray bottle
- Shake well before each use
- Spray onto damp hair and scalp, massaging gently
- Leave on for 510 minutes
- Rinse thoroughly

Benefits:

- Removes product buildup
- Balances scalp pH
- Leaves hair feeling fresh and clean

Tips:

- Use once a month for clarifying
- Avoid sun exposure after use due to lemon juice

CASTOR OIL AND SHEA BUTTER DEEP TREATMENT

Ingr:

- 2 Tbls castor oil
- 2 Tbls shea butter
- 1 Tbls argan oil

Proc:

- Melt shea butter in a double boiler until smooth
- Remove from heat and stir in castor oil and argan oil
- Apply to damp hair, focusing on the ends
- Leave on for 3045 minutes
- Rinse thoroughly

Benefits:

- Deeply nourishes and strengthens hair
- Restores shine and softness
- Repairs split ends

Tips:

- Use once a month for deep conditioning
- Cover hair with a warm towel for better absorption

ROSEMARY CASTOR OIL HOT OIL TREATMENT

Ingr:

- 2 Tbls castor oil
- 2 Tbls olive oil
- 10 drops rosemary essential oil

Proc:

- Mix castor oil, olive oil, and rosemary essential oil in a heatsafe bowl
- Warm the mixture in a microwave for 2030 seconds
- Apply to damp hair and scalp, massaging gently
- Cover with a shower cap and leave on for 30 minutes
- Rinse thoroughly

Benefits:

- Promotes hair growth
- Strengthens and nourishes hair
- Adds shine and softness

Tips:

- Use once a week for best results
- Test the oil temperature before applying to avoid burns

CASTOR OIL AND HONEY HAIR GLAZE

Ingr:

- 2 Tbls castor oil
- 1 Tbls honey
- 1 Tbls apple cider vinegar

Proc:

- Combine castor oil, honey, and apple cider vinegar in a bowl
- Mix well until fully blended
- Apply to damp hair from roots to ends
- Leave on for 20 minutes
- Rinse thoroughly

Benefits:

- Adds shine and smoothness
- Seals hair cuticles
- Reduces frizz

Tips:

- Use once every two weeks for a glossy finish
- Store in a cool, dry place to maintain consistency

MINT CASTOR OIL SCALP TONIC

Ingr:

- 2 Tbls castor oil
- 10 drops peppermint essential oil
- 1 Tbls witch hazel

Proc:

- Mix castor oil, peppermint essential oil, and witch hazel in a spray bottle
- Shake well before each use
- Spray onto the scalp and massage gently
- Leave on for 1015 minutes
- Rinse thoroughly

Benefits:

- Stimulates the scalp
- Reduces dandruff and itchiness
- Promotes healthy hair growth

Tips:

- Use twice a week for best results
- Store in a cool, dark place to preserve potency

CASTOR OIL EGG PROTEIN TREATMENT

Ingr:

- 2 Tbls castor oil
- 1 egg yolk
- 1 Tbls olive oil

Proc:

- Beat the egg yolk in a bowl until smooth
- Add castor oil and olive oil, mixing well
- Apply to damp hair and cover with a shower cap
- Leave on for 2030 minutes
- Rinse thoroughly with cool water

Benefits:

- Strengthens and repairs damaged hair
- Adds shine and softness
- Provides a natural protein boost

Tips:

- Use once a month for best results
- Rinse with cool water to avoid cooking the egg

5.3 PERSONALIZED BEAUTY ENHANCEMENTS

CASTOR OIL LIP PLUMPER

Ingr:

- 1 tsp castor oil
- 1 tsp cinnamon oil
- 1 Tbls beeswax

Proc:

- Melt beeswax in a double boiler until smooth
- Remove from heat and stir in castor oil and cinnamon oil until well blended
- Pour into a small container and let it cool to solidify

Benefits:

- Naturally plumps lips
- Adds shine and moisture
- Provides a subtle, pleasant tingling sensation

Tips:

- Apply as needed for a natural lip enhancement
- Store in a cool, dry place

CASTOR OIL BROW ENHANCER

Ingr:

- 1 Tbls castor oil
- 1 Tbls aloe vera gel
- 5 drops rosemary essential oil

Proc:

- Mix castor oil, aloe vera gel, and rosemary essential oil in a small bowl until well combined
- Apply to brows with a clean mascara wand or cotton swab before bed

Benefits:

- Promotes thicker and fuller brows
- Conditions and strengthens hair
- Encourages natural brow growth

Tips:

- Use nightly for best results
- Store in a cool, dark place

BRIGHTENING CASTOR OIL EYE SERUM

Ingr:

- 1 Tbls castor oil
- 1 tsp almond oil
- 5 drops vitamin E oil

Proc:

- Combine castor oil, almond oil, and vitamin E oil in a small dropper bottle
- Shake well to blend
- Apply a small amount around the eye area, tapping gently with fingertips

Benefits:

- Reduces dark circles and puffiness
- Hydrates and firms delicate skin
- Provides antiaging benefits

Tips:

- Use nightly before bed
- Be gentle when applying to avoid pulling the skin

CASTOR OIL BODY SHIMMER

Ingr:

- 1 Tbls castor oil
- 1 Tbls jojoba oil
- 1 tsp cosmetic grade shimmer powder

Proc:

- Mix castor oil, jojoba oil, and shimmer powder in a small bowl until well combined
- Apply to the body for a radiant glow
- Rub in gently until evenly distributed

Benefits:

- Provides a natural, radiant glow
- Hydrates and nourishes the skin
- Perfect for special occasions

Tips:

- Use as needed for a subtle shimmer
- Choose shimmer powder that matches your skin tone

CASTOR OIL CUTICLE CONDITIONER

Ingr:

- 1 Tbls castor oil
- 1 tsp coconut oil
- 5 drops lavender essential oil

Proc:

- Mix castor oil, coconut oil, and lavender essential oil in a small bowl until well combined
- Apply to cuticles and nails, massaging gently
- Leave on overnight or for at least 30 minutes

Benefits:

- Strengthens and conditions nails
- Softens and nourishes cuticles
- Promotes healthy nail growth

Tips:

- Use daily for best results
- Store in a cool, dry place

CASTOR OIL HIGHLIGHTER BALM

Ingr:

- 1 Tbls castor oil
- 1 tsp shea butter
- 1 tsp mica powder

Proc:

- Melt shea butter in a double boiler until smooth
- Remove from heat and stir in castor oil and mica powder until well blended
- Pour into a small container and let it cool to solidify

Benefits:

- Adds a natural highlight to cheekbones and brow bones
- Hydrates and nourishes the skin
- Provides a subtle, dewy glow

Tips:

- Apply to high points of the face as needed
- Choose mica powder that complements your skin tone

CASTOR OIL TINTED LIP BALM

Ingr:

- 1 Tbls castor oil
- 1 tsp beetroot powder
- 1 Tbls shea butter

Proc:

- Melt shea butter in a double boiler until smooth
- Remove from heat and stir in castor oil and beetroot powder until well blended
- Pour into a small container and let it cool to solidify

Benefits:

- Adds a natural tint to lips
- Hydrates and protects
- Provides a subtle, rosy color

Tips:

- Apply as needed for a natural lip color
- Store in a cool, dry place to maintain consistency

CASTOR OIL BLUSH TINT

Ingr:

- 1 Tbls castor oil
- 1 tsp rose petal powder
- 1 Tbls shea butter

Proc:

- Melt shea butter in a double boiler until smooth
- Remove from heat and stir in castor oil and rose petal powder until well blended
- Pour into a small container and let it cool to solidify

Benefits:

- Adds a natural flush to cheeks
- Hydrates and nourishes the skin
- Provides a subtle, rosy glow

Tips:

- Apply to cheeks as needed for a natural blush
- Store in a cool, dry place to maintain consistency

CASTOR OIL MAKEUP REMOVER

Ingr:

- 1 Tbls castor oil
- 1 Tbls olive oil
- 1 Tbls witch hazel

Proc:

- Combine castor oil, olive oil, and witch hazel in a small bottle
- Shake well to blend
- Apply to a cotton pad and gently wipe away makeup

Benefits:

- Effectively removes makeup
- Hydrates and nourishes the skin
- Leaves skin feeling clean and refreshed

Tips:

- Use nightly to remove makeup
- Store in a cool, dark place

CASTOR OIL HAIR PERFUME

Ingr:

- 1 Tbls castor oil
- 1 Tbls distilled water
- 10 drops essential oil of choice

Proc:

- Mix castor oil, distilled water, and essential oil in a small spray bottle
- Shake well before each use
- Spray lightly onto hair for a refreshing scent

Benefits:

- Adds a pleasant fragrance to hair
- Hydrates and nourishes
- Provides a light, nongreasy shine

Tips:

- Use as needed for a fresh scent
- Choose essential oils that complement your personal fragrance preference

BOOK 3: "HOLISTIC WELLBEING WITH CASTOR OIL: NATURE'S ELIXIR FOR A BALANCED LIFE"

CHAPTER 1: MIND AND EMOTIONAL HEALTH

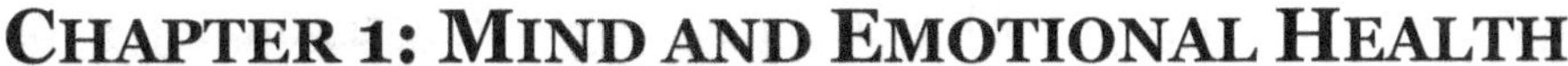

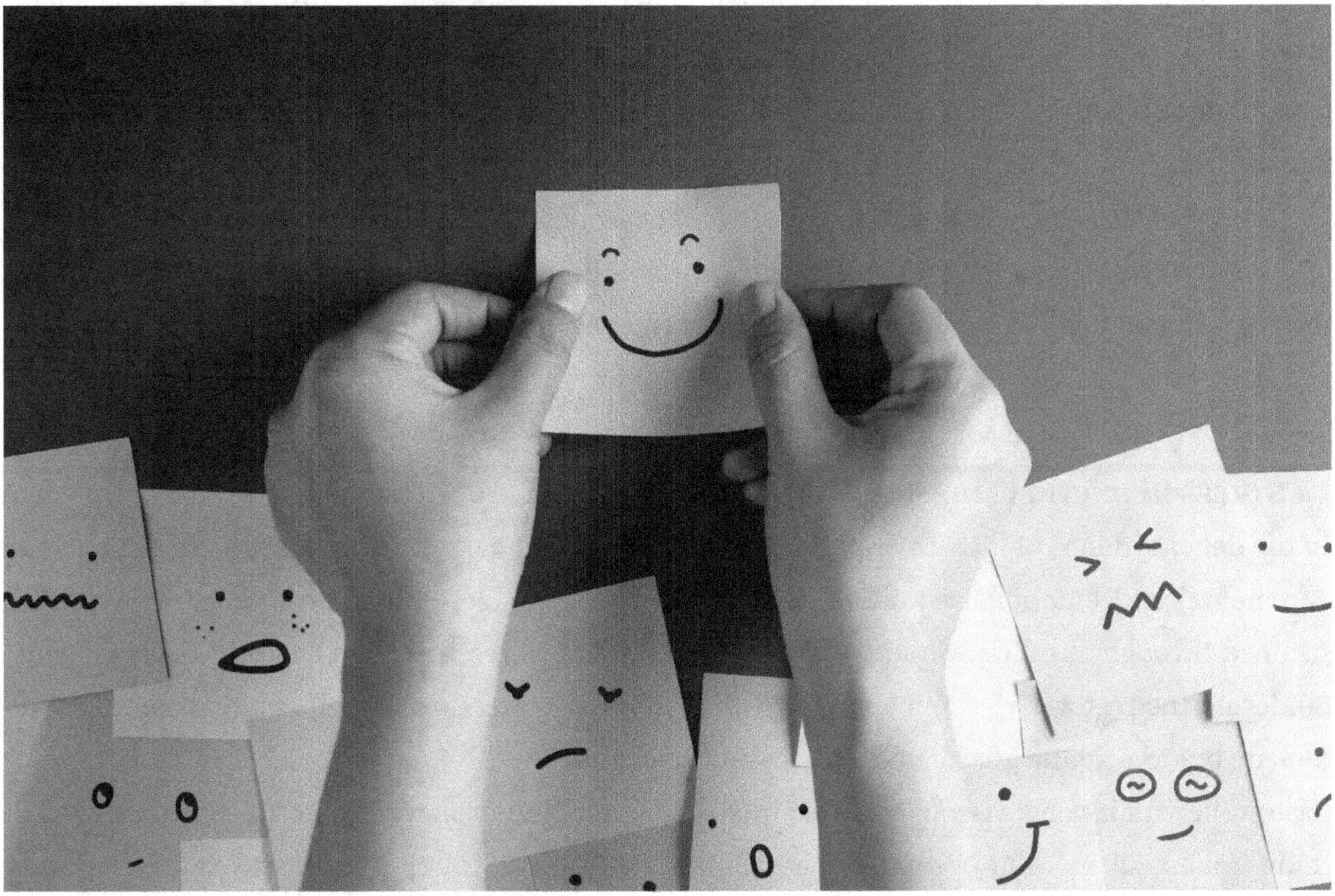

In the bustling rhythm of today's world, where the noise of constant connectivity often drowns out our inner peace, rediscovering tranquility can seem like a quest for a lost art. However, nestled within nature's bosom lies an elixir not just for the body but for the mind and spirit—castor oil, a humble yet powerful ally in the pursuit of mental and emotional health.

Imagine, if you will, a moment of pure serenity. It's early morning, and you are in the comfort of your living space, easing into a day that promises the usual stress, yet today feels different. You've decided to start with a simple ritual: a gentle massage of castis*JPG*oil on your temples, breathed in slowly to awaken senses dulled by sleep and calm a mind fraught with the clutter of unsorted dreams and pending tasks. This is not just a daily routine but a transformative practice that harnesses castor oil's potent properties to enhance mood and alleviate stress.

This chapter delves into how castor oil, a staple in traditional medicine cabinets for its physical healing attributes, becomes a gateway to emotional resilience and mental clarity.

The link between physical touch and emotional wellbeing is ancient and intuitive. When castor oil meets skin, it's not just a physical interaction but an emotional dance that soothes nerves and refreshes spirits. Aromatic compounds within the oil heighten this sensory experience, guiding you towards a palpable sense of calm.

Throughout the narratives and insights shared here, we journey through personal anecdotes and tangible, lifeenhanced stories from individuals who have woven castor oil into their mental health practices. You will learn not only about the biochemical properties that make castor oil a vital component of natural mental health care but also how to incorporate it into your daily routine to fight anxiety, promote better sleep, and ultimately, fortify your emotional resilience.

By the end of this chapter, castor oil will no longer be just another item in your wellness toolbox but a cherished companion on your journey towards holistic wellbeing, proving that sometimes, the path to mental clarity and emotional strength is as simple as reconnecting with the natural world.

1.1 STRESS REDUCTION AND SLEEP AID

In the delicate dance of life, stress and sleep are intertwined partners whose balance is crucial for our mental and emotional equilibrium. The nights when sleep is elusive can leave us feeling strained through our days, while the burdens of our daily stressors often chase us into our beds, hindering the restorative slumber we so desperately seek. Here, castor oil emerges not just as a remedy but as a gentle guardian of our nightly peace.

Castor oil, with its rich, viscous texture and deep histological properties, has long been revered in traditional medicine. But beyond its physical healing powers, it holds secrets to easing the mind and encouraging profound relaxation. The journey of castor oil's efficacy begins with its high concentration of ricinoleic acid, a remarkable antiinflammatory agent. When massaged into the skin, it doesn't just soothe the surface but penetrates deeply, promoting blood circulation and the soothing of nerves. This biological pathway lights the first beacon of relaxation, signaling the body to transition from the alertness of day to the peaceful descent into night.

The use of castor oil as a stress reducer and sleep aid can be visualized through the story of Elena, a middleaged nurse with two kids, grappling with the chaotic shifts of the healthcare sector. Her evenings were marred with restless thoughts, and sleep was but a fleeting visitor. Upon a friend's suggestion, Elena began incorporating castor oil into her nightly routine. She would warm a small amount of oil and gently massage it onto her forehead, temples, and the nape of her neck. The simple act of massaging created a meditative state, while the therapeutic properties of the oil worked their silent magic.

Over weeks, her sleep quality improved, and her days felt less burdensome. Elena's rejuvenation is a testament to how ancient remedies can bridge the gap to modernday stressors, offering solace in their enduring wisdom.

Exploring further the neuropsychological effects, researchers suggest that the sensory experience of touching and smelling castor oil can trigger a cascade of positive emotional responses. The physical touch involved in massaging the oil mimics a therapeutic act, activating the body's parasympathetic nervous system, which promotes rest and digest responses. The psychology of smell, too, plays into this, as the mild, earthy aroma of castor oil can be grounding, reducing feelings of anxiety and elevating mood.

Intriguingly, the benefits of castor oil extend into the realm of sleep not just through direct application but through the creation of a presleep ritual. Rituals, as structured repetitive actions, are powerful tools in signaling the brain that it's time to wind down. The act of massaging with castor oil, therefore, becomes more than skincare—it is a signal to the body to prepare for rest, creating a psychological readiness for sleep.

For those curious about optimizing their sleep environment alongside castor oil use, consider the ambiance of your sleep space. Combining the oil routine with elements like dimmed lights, soft bed linens, and a cool room temperature can enhance the overall effect. This holistic approach addresses not just the physical but also the environmental and sensory aspects that contribute to good sleep hygiene.

As we wrap up this exploration, it's vital to acknowledge that while castor oil presents a natural pathway to stress reduction and improved sleep, its integration into daily routines should be thoughtful and personalized. Each individual's response to therapies can vary, and the journey to discovering what works best for your unique constitution is both personal and profound.

Castor oil, therefore, is not just an agent of healing but a companion in your nightly journey to tranquility. Its use as a stress reducer and sleep aid is a testament to nature's capacity to nurture our most fundamental needs. In the embrace of its rich, soothing texture, may you find the peace that paves the way to restful nights and resilient days, proving once again that sometimes, the simplest remedies are the most profound.

1.2 ANXIETY RELIEF USING AROMATHERAPY

Imagine stepping into a serene sanctuary where the air itself seems imbued with calm; this is the potential of castor oil when utilized within the realm of aromathertherapy for anxiety relief. In the age where the word 'anxiety' finds its place in everyday vocabularies more often than we wish, natural therapeutics like aromatherapy offer a comforting hand back to inner tranquility.

Castor oil, though not typically heralded for its scent, forms a vital base to which other essential oils might be added, enhancing both efficacy and aroma. This approach to anxiety relief revolves around the holistic interaction between our olfactory senses and the emotional centers of the brain. A whiff of a calming scent can reroute the anxious energies, paving the way toward relaxation.

Take, for instance, the tale of Maria, a young graphic designer who found herself wrestling with tight deadlines and client demands. Her anxiety was palpable, a constant companion that drained her vibrant spirit. The turning point came when she attended a workshop on natural wellness, where she learned about the soothing synergy of castor oil mixed with lavender and chamomile. Every evening, Maria began to heat a small mixture of these oils to diffuse in her apartment. The effect was subtle at first but profound over time. The scent enveloped her in a cocoon of calm, easing her into a state of relaxation that she hadn't felt in years.

What Maria experienced was the power of scents in activating the limbic system, the brain's emotional powerhouse.

The molecules inhaled during aromatherapy interact directly with the amygdala and hippocampus, which are involved in emotion and memory. It is this interaction that can mitigate anxiety, rendering scents a powerful ally in the quest for peace.

Furthermore, the practice of using castor oil in aromatherapy transcends mere inhalation. When combined with massage, the physical act of rubbing the oil into the skin amplifies its benefits.

This is because the methodical action of massage is in itself a way to reduce psychological stress and improve emotional health. It stimulates the release of endorphins, often referred to as 'feelgood' hormones, which act as natural stress relievers.

Beyond personal anecdote, the scientific community has begun to take a keen interest in the validity of such holistic treatments. Research indicates that patients undergoing aromatherapy have shown significant reductions in anxiety levels, comparable in some cases to those observed with pharmaceutical interventions. These findings suggest not just the effectiveness but also the necessity of considering more integrative approaches to mental health care.

Expanding on the use of castor oil in aromatherapy, one must consider the environment conducive to such a practice. Creating a dedicated space for relaxation—be it a small corner of a room with soft lighting, comfortable seating, and perhaps a collection of soothing music—can enhance the therapeutic effects of aromatherapy. It's about crafting an atmosphere that supports wellness in every breath.

Moreover, it encourages those interested to engage actively with their treatment processes. The act of selecting oils, preparing blends, and setting the environment for aromatherapy can itself be incredibly empowering for individuals dealing with anxiety. It offers a sense of control over one's healing journey and an intimate connection with the process of selfcare.

In conclusion, while anxiety is a complex and multifaceted issue, the use of castor oil in aromatherapy presents a pathway filled with hope and healing. It's a testament to the power of natural remedies and their role in modern therapies. As we continue to explore and validate these ancient practices with contemporary science, we pave the way for a more holistic approach to mental health that honors the intricate connections between mind, body, and spirit.

Thus, whether you are like Maria, seeking solace from the noise of your daily grind, or simply someone curious about the natural paths to wellness, remember that sometimes, the most profound healing can begin with the simplest of scents breathed in a quiet moment.

1.3 MOOD ENHANCEMENT WITH CASTOR OIL

Within the colorful tapestry of our daily lives, our moods are the threads that give vibrancy and color to our existence. Just like a painter uses oils for their art, castor oil can be used to artfully enhance our mood, painting over the dull greys of depression and anxiety with brighter, more radiant hues.

Imagine embarking on a journey where each step you take lightens your spirits and soothes your mind.

This isn't just a daydream but a reality for those who discover the moodenhancing properties of castor oil. This natural elixir, derived from the humble castor bean, contains elements that not only heal the body but elevate the spirit.

Take Simon, for instance, a teacher who felt overwhelmed by the stresses of his highdemand job. His story reflects a common narrative in today's fastpaced world, where keeping up can sometimes mean tripping over our own feet. Simon's transformation began when he was introduced to castor oil during a wellness retreat focused on natural healing solutions. Intrigued by its therapeutic potential, he started applying a mixture of castor oil with a few drops of lemon essential oil to his wrists and temples each morning. It wasn't long before he noticed a subtle yet significant lift in his spirits. The ritual itself became a moment of selfcare that not only enhanced his mood but also empowered him to face the day with renewed optimism.

Simon's experience underscores the potent psychological impact of castor oil when combined with elements of aromatherapy. Scientific studies suggest that the fatty acids in castor oil may help stabilize mood by promoting healthy neurological function.

Ricinoleic acid, a major component of castor oil, plays a role in this by influencing neurotransmitter release, which can have a stabilizing effect on mood.

Moreover, the sensation of applying oil can be incredibly grounding, providing a physical connection to the earth that many of us lack in our digital, fastpaced environments. This physical act of massaging the oil gently into the skin stimulates the production of endorphins, known as the body's natural mood elevators. Through this tactile interaction, not only is the skin nourished but so is the soul, reinforcing the body's natural resilience against emotional disturbances.

Additionally, integrating castor oil into routine wellbeing practices can help establish a rhythm of selfcare that many find calming and uplifting. This was certainly the case for Nadia, a freelance writer battling seasonal affective disorder. Her adaptation of a morning routine including castor oil not only brightened her skin but also her outlook on dreary winter days. Nadia's mornings transformed from sluggish to invigorating, showing just how transformative simple additions to our daily routines can be for our mental health.

The versatility of castor oil extends beyond personal care to become a conduit for creating an environment conducive to positive mood enhancement. For instance, adding castor oil to a warm bath can amplify the therapeutic effects of water therapy, known for its relaxing and moodstabilizing benefits. The oil's rich texture and the warmth of the water work in tandem to create a sensory experience that can wash away the blues, leaving behind a sense of peace and contentment.

This approach to mood enhancement isn't just about combating negative feelings but about fostering a sustainable practice that enhances life's quality daily. It's about transforming routine into ritual, where the simple act of applying oil becomes a statement of intent to live life more joyfully and with greater emotional freedom.

In conclusion, while mood fluctuations are a natural part of human experience, managing them with natural aids like castor oil offers a harmonious path to maintaining emotional balance. The stories of Simon and Nadia are just two in a myriad of testimonials that celebrate the efficacy of castan oil not just as a supplement, but as a staple in the pursuit of enhanced wellbeing.

In embracing such natural solutions, we not only advocate for healthier lifestyles but also reconnect with the ageold wisdom that views nature as the greatest healer. In each drop of castor oil lies the potential for renewal, a reminder that within the grasp of our own hands lies the power to change our lives, one moodenhancing moment at a time. Through these practices, we weave a new thread in our tapestry, bright and strong, reflecting our commitment to live each day as fully and vibrantly as possible.

CHAPTER 2: HOUSEHOLD USES OF CASTOR OIL

In the sanctuary of home, where comfort meets practicality, the versatility of castor oil unfolds as a remarkable natural ally. Beyond its wellknown health and beauty benefits, this vibrant, golden elixir extends its utility into the very essence of domestic life. Embracing a sustainable lifestyle often begins with the small, everyday choices we make, from the cleaning products we use to the way we care for our belongings.

Imagine a typical weekend at home: You're faced with a long todo list that includes cleaning the kitchen, polishing furniture, and perhaps even tackling some garden pests that have been a bit too enthusiastic about your herbs. Now, picture achieving all these with a singular, ecofriendly ingredient—castor oil. Intriguing, isn't it?

Our journey through this chapter is about rediscovering simplicity and safety in household maintenance. Castor oil, a humble yet powerful extract, offers a myriad of applications that not only promise effectiveness but also care for the health of your family and the environment.

For instance, consider the peace of mind that comes from using a completely natural cleaning agent, one devoid of harsh chemicals, yet potent enough to cleanse and purify your living space. Or the satisfaction of preserving the luster of your wooden furniture with a substance that is as nurturing as it is polishing. These applications of castor oil not only serve practical purposes but also align with a conscious choice towards a more sustainable and toxinfree lifestyle.

The transition to incorporating castoid oil into your home care practices reflects a broader commitment to holistic living—connecting the dots between personal health, the wellbeing of your loved ones, and the overall impact on our planet. Throughout this chapter, we will explore these aspects, illustrating not just the 'how' but also the 'why' behind each use, turning everyday chores into acts of environmental stewardology and personal health advocacy. As we delve into these uses, let us appreciate the potency nestled within each drop of castor oil—a true testament to nature's generosity and a step forward in our collective journey towards an ecoconscious life.

2.1 NATURAL CLEANING SOLUTIONS

Embarking on the path of using castor oil as a cornerstone in household cleaning, we pivot towards simplicity and sustainability, steering clear of chemicalladen solutions that are commonplace in our stores. This subchapter unfolds the untapped potential of castor oil, not merely as a product but as a steadfast companion in your pursuit of a harmonious and healthy home.

In a world where our senses are constantly bombarded by the aggressive fumes of synthetic cleansers, imagine the solace found in the subtle, nutty aroma of castor oil blended into a cleaning solution that's both effective and safe.

Each application not only cleanses and purifies but also infuses your living space with the essence of nature's kindness.

Initiating this transition often begins with awareness. A study highlighting the adverse effects of common household chemicals on indoor air quality throws light on the urgent need for alternatives that do not compromise our health. Castor oil emerges as a beacon in this regard. Known for its antimicrobial properties, it serves as the backbone for crafting cleaning solutions that are both gentle and potent.

Consider the process of cleaning your kitchen, where residues of cooking oils and spices often leave behind a challenging mess. A concoction utilizing castor oil can adeptly break down greasy films without the harshness of synthetic degreasers, ensuring the surfaces are pristine and maintaining the integrity of your kitchen's ambiance.

Additionally, windows and glass surfaces that require a clear, streakfree finish benefit immensely from castor oilbased cleaners. The oil's unique properties prevent the smudging and accumulation of dust particles, rendering a clarity that enhances the influx of natural light into your rooms.

Moving beyond the kitchen, castor oil finds its place in the sanctity of the living area, where furniture, a repository of memories and comfort, demands care. Here, castor oil doubles as a polishing agent, safeguarding the wood while imparting a rejuvenating gloss that extends the life of each piece. This method not only preserves your furniture but does so by embracing an approach that's devoid of volatile organic compounds often found in commercial polishes.

In bathrooms, where cleanliness equates to wellness, the antifungal attributes of castor oil are particularly beneficial. Regular cleaning with solutions containing castor oil can help mitigate the formation of mold and mildew, common challenges in moisturerich environments, thereby safeguarding the health of your family.

The usage of castor oil extends into the realm of fabric care too. Delicate garments and linen can be washed using a mild detergent boosted with castor oil, ensuring thorough cleansing without compromising the fabric's integrity. This method is particularly advantageous for those with sensitive skin as it avoids the irritants commonly associated with laundry detergents.

Throughout these applications, the emphasis remains on integrating castor oil seamlessly into routine cleaning tasks, transforming them from mundane chores into acts of environmental stewardship and personal health care.

Each swipe of a cloth dampened with a castor oilinfused cleaner not only cleans but also reaffirms your commitment to a lifestyle that respects both personal wellbeing and the environment.

Moreover, the practice of using castor oil in home cleaning routines exemplifies a broader philosophy of living in alignment with nature's rhythms. It encourages a mindful approach, where choices are guided by their longterm impact on health and the planet. This conscious shift is reflective of a growing trend towards sustainable living that harmonizes modern needs with ecological responsibility.

Engaging with castor oil in this way also fosters a deeper connection with the origins and processing of the products we bring into our homes. Opting for coldpressed, hexanefree castor oil ensures that the ecological footprint of your cleaning regimen is minimal, aligning with principles of ethical sourcing and consumption.

As we conclude this exploration of castabout in domestic cleaning, it becomes evident that castor oil's role transcends its initial therapeutic and beauty applications. By adopting castor oil in our cleaning routines, we advocate for a life that is not only cleaner but also inherently richer, drawing ever closer to the ideals of health and harmony that castor oil so eloquently embodies.

2.2 PROTECTING AND POLISHING WOOD

In the cherished spaces we call home, wood forms an essential part of our surroundings, from eloquent hardwood floors to rugged oak cabinets and delicate antique furnishings. The rich, warm, inviting nature of wood can transform any room into a place of comfort and style. However, the beauty of wood does not maintain itself—it requires care and protection to preserve its luster and longevity. Herein lies the role of castor oil, a natural substance whose qualities extend beyond health remedies and beauty treatments to the realms of wood care.

Wood, by its nature, is susceptible to damage from environmental factors such as humidity, temperature changes, and wear from everyday use. Often, the products available for wood care are laden with harsh chemicals. These can offer a temporary sheen but might contribute to longterm damage including drying out or corroding the wood fibers. Contrary to these, castor oil provides a natural, effective alternative that not only improves the appearance of wood but also nourishes and protects it.

Utilizing castor oil for wood care involves recognizing its unique properties. The oil is rich in ricinoleic acid, a monounsaturated fatty acid, which acts as a natural humectant. This means it can attract and retain moisture, which is crucial for keeping wood hydrated and preventing it from becoming dry and brittle. Moreover, the viscosity of castor oil forms a protective layer over wood surfaces, shielding them from dust, dirt, and minor abrasives that can cause surface scratches.

Envision treating a cherished wooden dining table: regular cleaning might rid it of contaminants but doesn't provide lasting protection against daily wear and tear.

A gentle rub with a soft cloth dabbed in a small amount of castor oil not only brings out the natural grain and color of the wood but also creates a barrier that enhances the wood's resistance to impacts and marring.

Moreover, by bolstering the innate strength of wood, castor oil also helps in reducing the wood's vulnerability to pests, such as termites and beetles, that thrive on untreated wood. These pests are less likely to attack wood that is wellmaintained and covered by a film of oil, which disrupts their ability to latch onto the wood fibers.

Transitioning to castor oil for wood care also speaks volumes about our environmental and health consciousness. In a world increasingly cluttered with synthetic products, choosing a natural oil over a solventbased synthetic protector reduces the emission of volatile organic compounds (VOCs), which are harmful to both indoor air quality and the broader environment.

But the adoption of castor oil in wood care is not just about what it does—it's about how it harmonizes with the philosophy of living sustainably. Incorporating castor oil into the routine care of wooden items or structures promotes an ethos of renewal and sustainability. It's about creating practices that nourish and rejuvenate rather than deplete and replace.

Integrating the use of castor oil into wood care routines reflects an appreciation for the materials that make up our living spaces and a commitment to preserving these resources. It's a mindful approach that considers not just the aesthetic or superficial aspect of wood care but looks deeply at how to sustain its intrinsic value and resilience over time.

Given wood's prominence in home construction and furnishing, adopting natural methods for its care can have farreaching impacts. Each application of castor oil is a step towards maintaining the functional integrity and beauty of our wood possessions while aligning household practices with broader environmental and health goals.

Thus, as we delve deeper into adopting castor oil for wood protection and polishing, we are not merely engaging in a routine of maintenance; we are partaking in a deeper ritual of preservation—of our cherished woodworks, our health, and the planet. This holistic approach transcends mere aesthetics, encompassing a comprehensive lifestyle choice that embraces the principles of natural living and sustainability. Whether for the antique mahogany bookshelf or the everyday pine tables, castor oil stands as a pillar of protection, nurturing the past and safeguarding the future.

In the quiet corners of our homes, beyond the wooden floors and beneath the lush garden beds, often lie undetected, unwanted guests: pests. From the stubborn ants marching one by one to the more formidable mice, managing these creatures is a perennial challenge. However, in our quest to protect our sanctuaries, how do we strike the balance between efficacy and ecology? Here, castor oil emerges not only as a beneficial ally for health and beauty but also as an effective agent in organic pest control.

The role of castor oil in managing household pests can be traced back to its intrinsic properties. It is the viscous, organic nature of the oil that makes it less appealing for many types of pests. Unlike conventional pest control solutions that often wield harsh chemicals posing risks to health and the environment, castor oil provides a safer, cleaner alternative. This alignment with ecological principles doesn't just resonate with our desire to live sustainably but also amplifies our effort to create safe, nontoxic living spaces.

Imagine, for a moment, the typical areas of a home vulnerable to invasions—such as kitchens, basements, and gardens. These are the spaces where the natural repellent properties of castor oil can be most beneficial. For instance, kitchen counters, often the site of ant trails, can be safeguarded with a subtle application of castor oil. The oil's natural scent acts as a deterrent, disrupting the scent trails ants follow, thus preventing their procession without resorting to deadly toxins.

Transitioning to the outdoors, the garden, a hotspot for a myriad of pests, reveals another dimension of castor oil's versatility. Common pests in gardens include moles and voles, which not only disrupt the beauty of the landscape but can also undermine the health of the soil and plants. Here, the employment of castor oil becomes a strategic move. Applied around the perimeter of a garden or near the tunnels of these creatures, castor oil can serve as an effective repulsive barrier. Its robust smell and taste, unpleasant to moles and voles, encourage these burrowers to seek other areas less offensive to their senses.

Furthermore, castor oil can contribute to an integrated pest management strategy when used in combination with other organic practices. For instance, companion planting, which involves growing certain types of plants that naturally repel specific pests, can be supplemented with strategic placements of castor oil around the garden. This not only enhances the effectiveness of such organic methods but also ensures that the garden remains a thriving, chemicalfree environment.

The role of castor oil extends to the lesserknown, yet equally critical area of flying insects. While it does not kill these pests, it can act as a barrier deterrent. Applications around windows and doors can reduce the appeal of these entry points, discouraging entry and infestation.

Moreover, the importance of castor oil in organic pest control reflects a broader commitment to health and environmental stewardship. Each application is an act of preservation—protecting not just our immediate surroundings but also contributing to a larger environmental impact. By choosing castor oil, homeowners can avoid the ecological footprint left by synthetic pesticides, which often permeate beyond their target areas to affect wildlife and water sources adversely.

In essence, adopting castor oil for pest control is not just about deterring unwelcome guests; it's about embracing a philosophy of living harmoniously within our environments. It underscores a commitment to approaches that respect the delicate balance of nature, ensuring that our homes remain sanctuaries for us without becoming fortresses against the natural world.

Through its multifaceted applications, castor oil champions an approach that is as compassionate as it is effective. As we integrate this natural oil into our pest management practices, we do more than merely protect our homes; we contribute to a legacy of sustainability. This not only reinforces the practice of safe, organic pest control but also aligns with our deeper values of care, conservation, and responsible stewardship of our planet. As such, castor oil stands not just as a tool, but as a testament to the power of natural solutions in our ongoing dialogue with nature.

Chapter 3: Castor Oil for Pet Care

In the quiet corners of our homes, where wagging tails and gentle purrs abound, our pets nuzzle their way into the very fabric of our families, bringing languid comfort and vibrant joy. It's in the soft gaze of our cats and the loyal eyes of our dogs that we often find a heartfelt connection quite unlike any other. But with the sweetness of their companionship comes the inevitable anxiety we bear over their wellbeing. Traditional pet care products, laden with chemicals, pose a silent question—could there be a more natural way to ensure the health and happiness of our furry friends?

Enter castor oil, nature's elixir, embraced not only for its impressive range of applications in human health and beauty but also for its remarkable benefits for pet care. Drawing from the same properties that make castor oil a staple in our wellness routines, it emerges as a potent ally in managing the health of pets. Its antibacterial and antifungal virtues make it an excellent choice for maintaining skin health, and its hydrating properties soothe dry paws and noses, ensuring our pets are not only healthy but also comfortable.

Consider a winter evening, as you notice your beloved pet's coat losing its luster or their paws cracking from the cold. Implementing a simple routine that includes a gentle massage with warm castor oil can transform these moments of concern into opportunities for bonding, turning routine care into a session of quiet connection. Such practices do more than soothe and heal; they deepen the trust and understanding between you and your pet, fostering a relationship grounded in care and attentiveness.

As we venture through this chapter, remember that every recommendation enhances the natural vitality of your pets, aligning with the rhythms of a life lived close to nature's heart. Castor oil is not just a bottle of oil; it's a testament to the gentle power of nature's care—a bridge between human intentions and animal needs, wrapped in the warmth of holistic health practices.

3.1 Safe Uses for Dogs and Cats

Nestled within the larger narrative of natural wellness, embracing castor oil for pet care reflects a burgeoning interest in leveraging nature's simplicity to foster health and comfort for our fourlegged family members. Dive into the heart of many pet owners' concerns, and you'll often find a compelling desire to nurture their dogs and cats in a safe, toxinfree environment. Castor oil, distinct for its therapeutic properties among humans, holds a treasure trove of applications for dogs and cats, too, when used with mindful preparation and attention to safety.

When contemplating the introduction of any new element into your pet's regimen, particularly one as potent as castor oil, the initial steps involve understanding its fundamental interactions with their unique biology. For both canine and feline companions, the primary benefit of castor oil lies in its ability to soothe skin irritations and fortify fur health. Its rich ricinoleic acid content, known for its antiinflammatory capabilities, makes it an astute choice for topical applications aimed at alleviating dry, itchy skin or promoting a glossy, vibrant coat.

Harnessing castor oil's benefits begins with a cautious approach, particularly in recognizing that what serves humans well doesn't automatically translate as safe for pets. A practical beginning is the patch test—applying a small amount on a less sensitive part of your pet's skin to observe any adverse reactions before committing to a regular regimen. This simple preliminary step helps ensure compatibility with your pet's skin, sidestepping potential irritants and setting the stage for a harmonious usage.

In discussing the topical utility, consider a common scenario: a dog with dry, flaky skin, especially amid winter's harshness, or a cat with patches of hair loss after a stressful move. Here, the soothing properties of castor oil can be gently massaged onto the affected areas, providing relief and aiding in the recovery of healthy skin and fur. However, adherence to nonoral usage is crucial. The digestive systems of dogs and cats do not process the same components as humans with the same efficacy, and the ingestion of castor oil can lead to distressing gastrointestinal reactions.

As much as castor oil serves as a balm for physical ailments, its integration into your pet care practices also weaves an emotional tapestry, enhancing the bond between pet and caregiver. Picture the weekly routine of gently massaging your cat or dog with a light blend of castor oil and a suitable carrier oil. This ritual doesn't just serve skin and fur; it develops a rhythm of care and trust, a reassurance to your furry companions that they are safe, loved, and cared for.

Yet, with its potent effects, the usage of castor oil must be navigated with an informed perspective, especially understanding what it isn't suitable for. It is not advisable, for instance, to use castor oil for internal ailments commonly found in pets, such as digestive issues, without professional vet consultation. Misuse can easily tilt the scale from beneficial to harmful, turning a healing intention into potential hazard.

Venturing beyond routine care, the occasional need to address parasites like ticks and fleas presents another dimension where castor oil might play a role. In these instances, its application should be specific, targeted, and always external. A diluted solution can be brushed through the fur, helping to loosen the grip of parasites, which can then be combed out, minimizing the use of chemicalladen products. This approach not only aligns with a natural product ethos but also reduces chemical exposure for both pet and owner.

The use of castor oil in pets' care also extends into holistic wellness practices, where its calming scent could complement aromatherapy sessions designed specifically for pets. These sessions, tailored to not overwhelm delicate animal senses, can help reduce anxiety and promote relaxation, especially in pets prone to nervousness or those recovering from illness or trauma.

Every narrative shared, every guideline offered, springs from a foundation of deepcare and respect for the nature of our pets. From the very onset, where a patch test initiates a journey into natural care, to the detailed, sensitive application avoiding ingestion, the story of castor oil in pet care is penned with an ink of caution and a script of affection. It's an ongoing dialogue, a consistent checkin with each pet's response, ensuring that this natural remedy enriches the lives of pets in a manner that's both safe and effective. In the grand tapestry that forms our lives with our pets, castor oil can be a single yet significant thread, woven with care to strengthen the bond and enhance the health of our beloved companions.

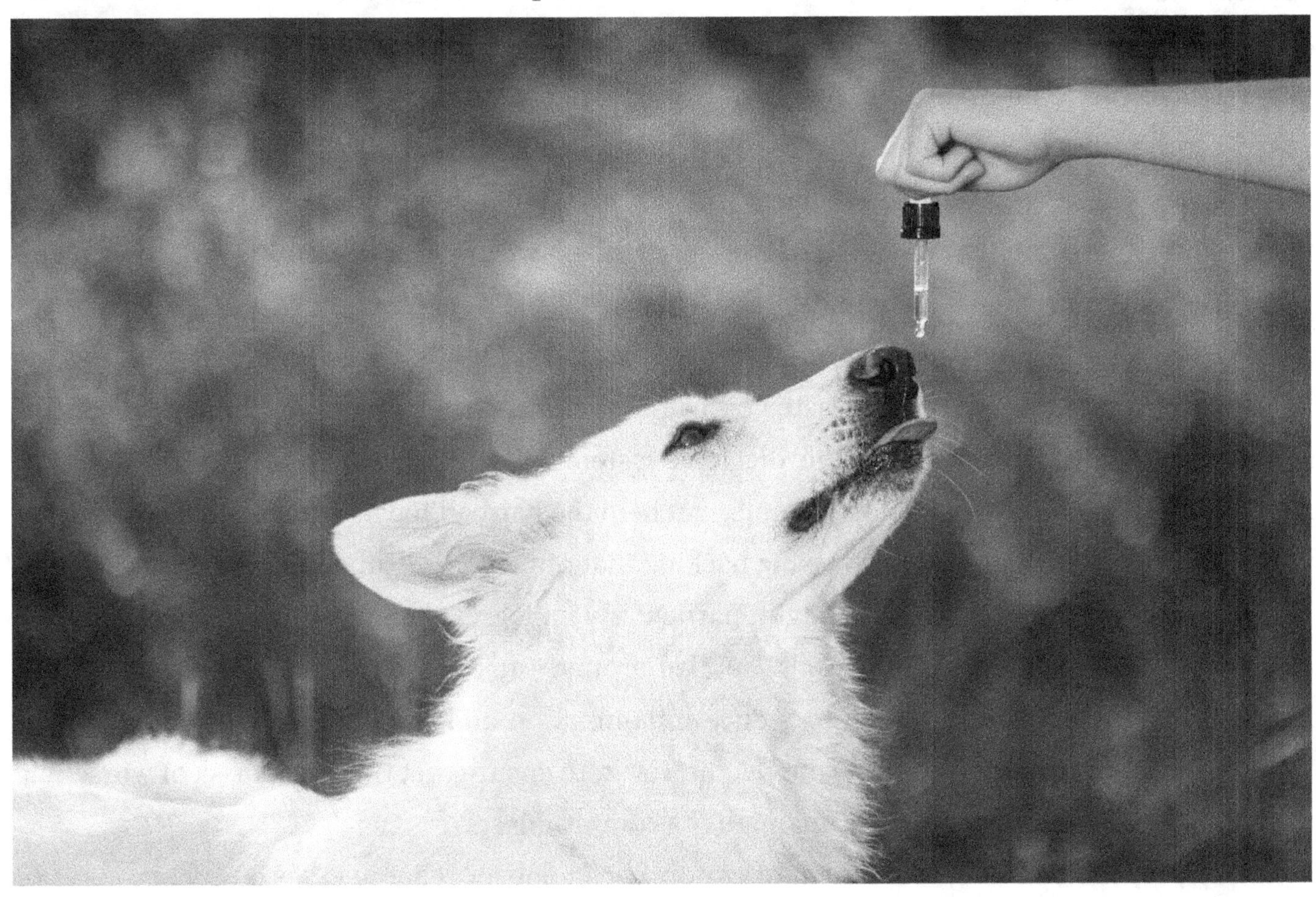

Anyone who has ever looked into the eyes of a beloved pet suffering from discomfort or illness knows the helpless feeling that accompanies the desire to provide relief. Whether it's a pesky skin irritation, a bout of ear mites, or those alltoocommon fur balls that plague our feline friends, pet owners often search for gentle, natural remedies. Castor oil, with its wide array of applications, stands out as a versatile ally in treating such common pet ailments, merging nature's kindness with healing efficacy.

At the outset, it's vital to embrace a holistic perspective, one that views the use of castor oil not as a cureall but as part of a broader approach to pet health. When considering its application for common pet ailments, understanding the specific condition is crucial. This not only ensures appropriate use of castor oil but also safeguards the health of the pet through a personalized approach to their care.

For instance, consider the frequent problem of skin irritations and rashes. The antiinflammatory properties of castor oil make it an excellent choice for soothing these discomforts. Apply a thin layer over the affected area can form part of a broader treatment plan, providing relief while other therapeutic actions take effect. Keeping in mind that the safety and comfort of the pet are paramount, it's essential to ensure that the area treated with castor oil remains inaccessible to licking, as ingestion could lead to undesirable effects.

Moving to a concern many cat owners face: hairballs. While not a remedy for preventing the ingestion of fur during grooming, castor oil can assist in the more comfortable passage of this indigestible material through the feline digestive system.

A minuscule dab on their paws, for example, can help the hairball navigate through the intestines more smoothly, alleviating the distressing hacking that often accompanies a hairball blockage.

Ear infections are another common plight, particularly in dogs. Owners might consider a mixture of castor oil with soothing herbs or oils, applied around the external part of the ear, but never inside the ear canal. This can help to reduce inflammation and discomfort associated with ear infections. It's important to consult your vet, however, to ensure that there is no risk of worsening the condition, especially if the eardrum might be compromised.

Moreover, the moisturizing component of castor oil can deliver relief in cases of dry paw pads or noses, a frequent concern during colder months. Applying a small amount to these areas can prevent cracking and bleeding, restoring moisture and elasticity. However, one must oversee the pet to prevent licking of the areas where the oil has been applied, to keep the ingestion to a minimum.

While each of these applications demonstrates the potential of castur oil in addressing specific ailments, it's imperative to remind pet owners that not all problems are suitable for home treatment. Professional veterinary advice should be sought in situations beyond minor ailments or where symptoms persist despite treatment. The role of castor oil should be seen as complementary, capable of providing relief as part of a wider, vetapproved treatment plan.

The narrative of using castor oil in pet care is also enriched by the stories of those who have found success with its judicious use. These anecdotes not only provide a blueprint for new users but also testify to the practical and gentle healing properties of castor oil when incorporated correctly into pet care routines. They underline the themes of empathy and caution, reinforcing that the wellbeing of the pet remains at the heart of all treatment choices.

Ultimately, integrating castor motor oil into treatments for common pet ailments embodies the convergence of affection, science, and nature. It exemplifies the approach that seeks to harmonize natural remedies with conventional veterinary science, promoting health and comfort without compromising safety. In this light, castor oil shines not merely as a substance but as a symbol of thoughtful, loving care that pet owners aspire to provide for their animal companions.

3.3 COAT AND PAW CARE

In the realm of pet care, the language of love is often spoken through the meticulous attention we pay to the health of our pets' coats and paws. These areas, while sometimes neglected in the daily hustle of life, are vital indicators of a pet's overall wellbeing and gateways to fostering a healthier, happier animal companion.

The integration of castor oil, a venerable and versatile gift from nature, into the care regimen for pet coats and paws, illuminates a path to nurturing these essential aspects with gentle, effective practices.

Imagine a brisk morning walk, our joyful companions at our side, paws padding softly alongside. The health of their paws is paramount, as these are not just the point of contact with the world but are as sensitive and prone to discomfort as our own hands and feet. Dry, cracked paw pads are not uncommon and can lead to discomfort and more serious complications if not addressed. Here, castor oil emerges as a soothing balm. Applied after a gentle cleaning of the paws, it can hydrate and heal, creating a barrier that protects against the ravages of salty roads in winter or hot pavements in summer. It's these small acts of wellbeing—like the careful application of a layer of castor oil—that strengthen the bond between pets and their families, turning routine care into a gesture of deep affection.

Transitioning from the paws to the coat, the benefits of castor oil continue to shine. A healthy, shining coat is not just a pleasure to behold but a mirror of a pet's internal health. Many pets suffer from itchy, dry skin or dull, brittle fur, symptoms often exacerbated by commercial grooming products laden with harsh chemicals. Integrating castor oil into your pet's grooming routine can change this narrative drastically. When massaged into the coat, its inherent properties help in moisturizing the skin beneath, easing dryness and dandruff, and imparting a natural luster to the fur. This application not only comforts the pet but also transforms their coat into a softer, more vibrant cloak that speaks to their improved health and vitality.

These applications, rich in practical benefit and narrative, transcend mere grooming; they act as agents of comfort and signals of care. The story of a rescued dog, perhaps with a dull coat and wary eyes, gradually transforming as the weeks pass, fur becoming glossy under the hands of a loving owner diligently applying castor oil—this is a testimony to the power of natural care. It illustrates not just a treatment of symptoms but a holistic enhancement of life quality.

For pet owners, however, the use of castor oil should be approached with informed caution. Proper application techniques ensure that the oil serves as a remedy rather than a nuisance or a hazard. A light amount, thoroughly rubbed into the coat or paw pads, suffices. Overapplication can lead to excessive greasiness, and the pet might attempt to lick it off, leading to the possible ingestion of too much oil. Here lies the importance of moderation and observation—a dual principle that governs the use of natural remedies in pet care.

In these narratives of healing and care, the bond between pets and their guardians grows deeper. Each stroke of the brush or rub of a towel becomes a moment of connection, a mutual understanding of comfort and caring.

It is in these quiet, often unseen interactions that the true value of castor oil in coat and paw care is revealed—not merely in the sheen of a wellgroomed coat or the softness of healed paws but in the shared moments of tenderness and wellbeing.

Thus, castor oil, in its application for pet coat and paw care, is not just contributing to the aesthetic appeal or physical health of pets. It becomes woven into their daily rituals, a symbol of the nurturing spirit of their caregivers. This alignment with natural methods strengthens as pet owners witness the transformation in their beloved companions, fueled not by harsh chemicals but by the purity and potency of nature itself. The journey with castor oil becomes a beautiful narrative of health, comfort, and caring, whispered in the joyful barks and contented purrs of animals who feel as cherished as they truly are.

CHAPTER 4: CASTOR OIL FOR THE GARDEN

As we explore the garden—a place of growth, nurturing, and nature's own alchemy—it becomes clear that our quest for a balanced life can flourish right in our own backyards. Castor oil, esteemed for its health and beauty benefits, also emerges as a marvel in the garden, a testament to the endlessly versatile powers of this cherished oil.

Imagine stepping into your garden, where the fragrances of blooming flowers mingle with the earth's rich aroma. Here, nature is at its most generous, offering us food, flowers, and a sanctuary of serene beauty. Yet, maintaining such a garden oasis can be as challenging as it is rewarding. It necessitates a harmony between growth and protection, sustenance, and sustainability. This is where castor oil steps in with its gentle, yet powerful capabilities.

This chapter is dedicated to those who see the garden not just as a place to cultivate plants, but as an opportunity to foster a sustainable, chemicalfree ecosystem that thrives season after season. Many gardeners struggle with the dilemma of repelling pests and nurturing plants in a way that doesn't rely on harsh chemicals. Castor oil, an ecofriendly solution, becomes a savior in this context. Its use as a natural fertilizer provides essential nutrients to the soil, enhancing the vitality of your plants. The oil can also be part of a pest control strategy that doesn't harm the earth or the creatures that benefit your garden's health.

Moreover, our connections with our gardens are deeply personal. They are spaces that heal, rejuvenate, and connect us with the elements. Integrating castor oil into your gardening practice not only enhances plant health but also aligns your outdoor space with your values of living cleanly and sustainably.

As we delve deeper into the uses of castor oil in the garden, we'll uncover how it helps in preventing plant diseases, serves as a natural fertilizer, and even the ways it can protect your garden's wooden structures. Each usage underscores a commitment to an ecofriendly lifestyle, making our green spaces not just a source of personal joy but also a beacon of environmental stewardness. Through this exploration, we discover that each drop of castor oil holds within it a promise of renewal, not just for our bodies, but for the earth itself.

4.1 FERTILIZER ALTERNATIVES WITH CASTOR OIL

In the verdant world of gardening, the quest for sustainable growth spurs endless innovation, leading us to rediscover ancient substances with modern applications. Castor oil, praised for its health benefits and protective qualities in skincare, also emerges as a remarkable ally in the garden—particularly as an ecofriendly alternative to traditional chemical fertilizers.

At the heart of every thriving garden is soil health. Just as the human body relies on vital nutrients, plants depend on the soil to provide them with the sustenance they need. However, many contemporary gardening practices, heavily dependent on synthetic fertilizers, have led to nutrient depletion, damaging the very foundation of plant health and reducing the soil's natural fertility. Castor oil presents a natural solution that not only nurtures the plants but also enhances the soil without the adverse effects associated with chemical treatments.

This natural elixir, derived from the seeds of the Ricinus communis plant, contains beneficial properties that make it an excellent choice for gardeners aiming to maintain soil health and promote plant growth organically. Its application to the soil helps in creating a healthier, more balanced soil ecosystem. When castor oil penetrates the soil, it encourages the presence of beneficial microbes. These microbes play a crucial role in nutrient cycling, breaking down organic matter, and making nutrients more accessible to plants. This process not only nourishes the plants but also strengthens them against diseases and pests.

Moreover, castor oil has unique properties that retain moisture in the soil. This feature is particularly beneficial in arid climates or during dry seasons, where water conservation is critical. By using castor oil in the soil, plants maintain hydration more efficiently, reducing the need for frequent watering and safeguarding the garden during times of drought.

Beyond its role in nurturing plant health, castor oil acts as a natural deterrent against soilborne pests. The oil's viscous nature forms a barrier that can prevent pest infestation, which is often exacerbated by the use of synthetic chemicals that disrupt the natural pest predators in the environment. Gardeners may observe a significant reduction in common garden pests, such as nematodes, which are known to damage root systems and stunt plant growth.

Despite these extensive benefits, integrating castor oil into your garden practices demands understanding and patience. Unlike synthetic quickfix solutions, the effectiveness of castic oil unfolds gradually, requiring regular application and a bit of faith in nature's own rhythms. It offers a shift towards slow gardening—a practice that aligns with the cycles of nature, rather than seeking to control or expedite them.

Imagine your garden as a microcosm of the natural world, a place where life cycles flow unimpeded by harsh chemicals. Here, flowers bloom a bit brighter, leaves grow a bit fuller, and all is interconnected. Each application of castor oil not only feeds the plants but also heals the earth, restoring a bit more of the natural harmony that modern practices have disrupted.

This gentle yet profound impact of castor oil sets a foundation for longterm health and sustainability. It creates a legacy in the garden—not just in the beauty of the plants and the yield of the crops but in the vitality of the soil itself.

As holistic health practitioners, we recognize the parallel between the wellbeing of our environment and our own health. Thus, integrating castilk oil into our gardening routine goes beyond mere plant care—it becomes an act of environmental stewardship, a step toward a more sustainable and healthful existence.

Transitioning to castor oil as a fertilizer alternative does not need to be overwhelming. Start small, perhaps with a single flower bed or a vegetable patch. Observe the changes in plant health and soil quality and adjust your practices as you learn from the garden itself. Over time, as you mix this ancient remedy with your soil, you may find that you're not just growing plants—you're cultivating a sanctuary for yourself and a testament to the regenerative power of nature.

Embracing castor oil in your gardening practice invites a deeper connection with the environment and a commitment to nurturing life in its purest forms. The journey toward a sustainable, chemicalfree garden using castic oil is not only about growing plants but about growing alongside them in knowledge, health, and harmony.

4.2 NATURAL PLANT DISEASE PREVENTION

In the everevolving dialogue between humans and nature, maintaining the health of our gardens is akin to nurturing our own bodies. Much like the noninvasive, holistic approaches we prefer for our health, plants thrive under the care of natural, gentle treatments. Herein lies the beauty of castor oil – a remedy drawn from the earth, offering a shield against plant diseases, enriching our quest for garden sustainability and health.

At the heart of natural plant disease prevention, the benefits of castor oil stem from its inherent fungicidal and antibacterial properties. These characteristics make it an excellent choice for gardeners who seek to manage plant diseases without resorting to harsh chemicals that can leech into the soil and beyond. By applying castor oil to the garden, we engage in a form of preventive care that is not only effective but aligns with an ethos of environmental responsibility and health.

The presence of ricinoleic acid, a key component of castro oil, plays a pivotal role in its ability to fend off disease. This unique compound has shown considerable efficacy in suppressing the growth of molds, mildew, and other fungi that typically afflict garden plants. Picture a garden where the leaves of tomatoes remain vibrantly green and the stems of roses are robust, free from the black spots of mildew. This vision is achievable with the regular use of castor oil as part of a holistic garden management plan.

Moreover, the use of castic oil encourages a symbiotic relationship with the beneficial microbes in the soil. These microbes are essential for a healthy garden ecosystem, aiding in nutrient absorption, decomposition, and even deterring pathogenic bacteria.

By nurturing these microbes rather than destroying them, castic oil helps create a natural barrier against many common garden diseases.

For any gardener, the words "plant disease" conjure a sense of dread. The disappointment of wilted leaves and the frustration of lost crops can dishearten the most passionate. However, integrating castic oil into regular garden care can significantly reduce these occurrences. It acts not just as a treatment, but more importantly, as a preventive measure, creating conditions less conducive to disease outbreaks.

Consider a typical scenario in any garden—cucumbers beginning to flourish next to lush tomatoes. Without protection, powdery mildew can quickly set in, especially in warmer climates or during damp, humid seasons. A prophylactic approach involving castor oil could involve treating the plants before the signs of disease manifest. Applied in the right concentration and frequency, the oil forms a protective layer that is inhospitable to the spores of fungi and other pathogens.

Moving beyond mere disease prevention, the inclusion of castric oil in garden care routine also offers an opportunity to connect with nature on a deeper level. As gardeners, the choice of castor oil transcends its functionality; it becomes a declaration of our values—values rooted in sustainability and the wellbeing of the ecosystem. This connection deepens our understanding and appreciation of the natural world, as we see our gardens not only survive but thrive under our care. While the application of castor oil offers numerous benefits, it is essential to approach its use mindfully. Every garden is unique, and the climate, soil type, and plant variety all play critical roles in how castor oil should be integrated into garden care. Observing the response of the garden to initial applications and adjusting accordingly ensures that the oil provides maximum benefit without causing harm. It's a delicate balance, driven by observation and adaptation, elements fundamental to successful gardening.

In practical terms, embracing castic oil for plant disease prevention also represents a step towards greater autonomy in garden management. By reducing reliance on commercial chemical products, gardeners can gain more control over what enters their environment and ultimately, what contributes to their harvests. This selfsufficiency not only enhances personal health and safety but also contributes to a larger movement towards environmental stewardship and sustainable living. As we continue to explore more profound ways to interact with our environment, using castor oil in the garden offers a simple, yet powerful, testament to what can be achieved when we align our gardening practices with the principles of nature and holistic health.

It invites us to imagine a world where gardens are not only beautiful and productive but are also vibrant ecosystems that mirror our commitment to health and sustainability.

In these gardens, every plant nurtured with castor oil stands as a leafy testament to the possibilities inherent in choosing natural, lifesupporting methods.

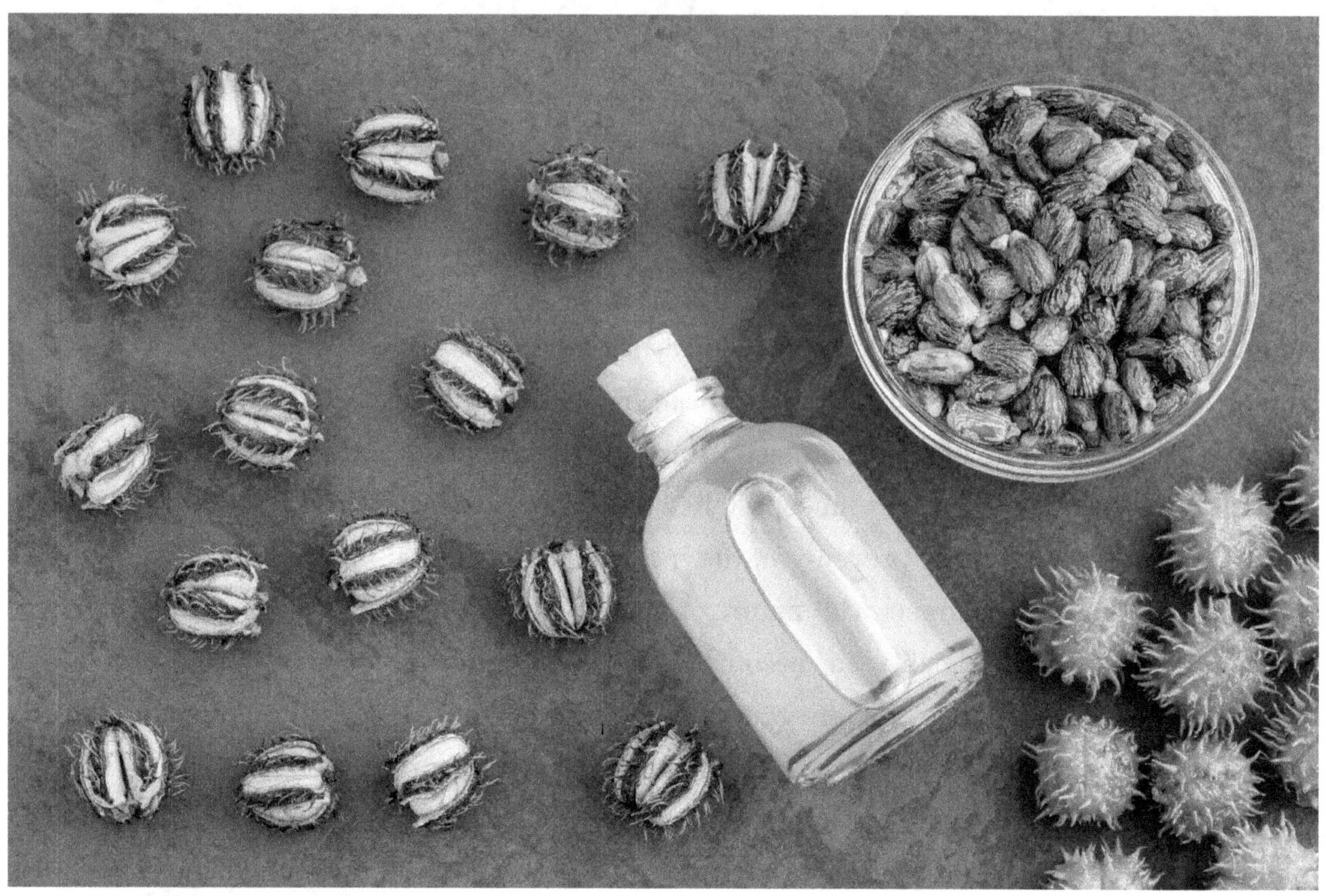

4.3 PEST REPELLENT RECIPES

In the garden, the delicate interplay between growth and guardian can often be disrupted by unwelcome guests—pests. Those small, industrious critters that nibble away at our carefully nurtured plants can cause a great deal of frustration for any gardener. But in our quest for harmony within the ecosystem of our gardens, a compassionate approach to pest control can be both effective and in alignment with our principles of natural care. Here, castor oil emerges not only as a protector of plants but as a safeguard that respects the delicate balance of our garden environments.

Using castor oil as a pest repellent is driven by a deeper understanding of nature's mechanisms. The oil's natural properties, which include its strong scent and thick texture, make it unappealing to many common garden pests such as moles, voles, and even insects. When introduced into the garden environment, it creates a barrier that is deterrent yet not destructive, offering a solution that preserves the wellbeing of both plants and the smaller creatures that might otherwise be harmed by more aggressive treatments.

Integrating castor oil into pest management routines speaks to a philosophy of prevention rather than eradication. The goal is to discourage pests from settling and feeding in the garden without resorting to measures that strip away the garden's natural resilience. For instance, the thick viscosity of castor oil helps in coating the leaves and stems of plants, creating a tactfully unpleasant surface for pests. This method is particularly effective in deterring insects that rely on their sense of taste and touch to navigate their feeding grounds.

Moreover, the scent of castor oil, while mild to human senses, is robust in the olfactory landscape of many garden pests. This can mask the enticing aromas of ripe vegetables and lush foliage, essentially cloaking the plants in an olfactory invisibility cloak. With regular application, the garden becomes a less attractive target, encouraging pests to move along without finding residence among your cherished plants.

Castor oil's role in natural pest control also extends to its biodegradable nature—beneficial for those who cultivate their gardens with the future of the planet in mind. Unlike synthetic pesticides that remain in the environment, potentially disrupting soil and water ecosystems, castor oil degrades naturally.

This degradation ensures that it doesn't accumulate within the garden biosphere, thus maintaining the integrity and health of the soil, which is crucial for sustainable gardening practices.

Those who integrate castor oil into their gardening strategy often find that it enhances their relationship with the natural world. It encourages a garden management style that respects life's complexities—recognizing that every creature, even those considered pests, has a role to play in the broader environmental scheme. This holistic approach doesn't just address the symptoms (the pests) but delves deeper into the garden's health, improving plant resilience and ecological balance.

Applying castor oil for pest repellence is a practice in patience and persistence. It is not an instantaneous solution but a progressive one. Success in using castor oil effectively requires understanding the patterns and behaviors of garden pests and adjusting applications based on seasonal changes and observed effectiveness. The process of trial and reflection fosters a deeper engagement with the garden, turning daily maintenance into a dialogue with nature.

Furthermore, employing castor oil in pest management contributes to a cycle of health that benefits the entire garden. Plants free from the stress of pests can invest more energy into growth and fruit production, which leads to robust harvests. Healthy plants are also better able to withstand diseases and adverse weather conditions, enhancing overall garden vitality.

Embracing castor oil as a pest repellent also illustrates a broader commitment to sustainable living. It's a testament to the principle that effective garden care can synchronize with environmental ethics, providing food and beauty without compromising the health of our planet. This method allows gardeners to cultivate not just plants but a legacy of respect and care for nature.

Whether you are a seasoned gardener or a beginner, integrating castor oil into your pest management regimen offers a way to protect your garden while honoring the ecological balance. It encourages a shift towards more conscious gardening practices, where every drop of oil used is a step towards more ethical, sustainable living. In adopting such practices, we garden not just for ourselves but for the world we inhabit, nurturing a patch of the earth that can inspire and flourish as a model of harmony and health.

DOWNLOAD YOUR BONUS

Castor Oil for Eco-Friendly Living

Sustainable Tips for a Greener Home and Lifestyle

Dear reader,

thank you for purchasing my book and downloading the bonus. I hope you get as much value from it as possible.

I would be immensely pleased to have your opinion through a review on Amazon.

Lots of love

Waverly Christie

CHAPTER 5: CREATIVE AND MISCELLANEOUS USES

As we journey deeper into the myriad uses of castor oil, uncovering its potential in health and beauty, an intriguing dimension unveils itself in this chapter. Here, we explore its creative and miscellaneous applications that promise to enrich our lives in unexpected ways. Perhaps it's the silken touch of castor oil that first hinted at its versatility, or the way it seamlessly integrates into various facets of daytoday activities, beckoning us to look beyond the conventional.

Imagine a lazy Sunday afternoon, a canvas awaiting your creative touch. Castor oil enters as an unsung hero in the arts, serving as a binder for pigments in homemade paints, offering that perfect consistency and a professional finish that enhances the vibrancy of colors. Artists, crafting their visions with strokes of brilliance, can find in castor oil an ally that not only brings their artwork to life but also preserves their masterpieces with its natural, enduring properties.

Transitioning from the palette to the stage of personal wellness practices, castor oil proves its mettle yet again. Incorporating small rituals, such as adding castor oil to meditation candles, not only extends their lifespan but also enhances the calming ambiance, supporting deeper relaxation and focus. Such rituals pave the way for a balanced life, rooting wellness in simplicity and sustainability.

Moreover, who would have thought that this same elixir could transform our living spaces? A dash of castor oil in your polishing arsenal can breathe new life into wooden heirlooms, protecting and giving them a lustrous sheen that speaks to the oil's protective qualities. This not only saves additional expenses on synthetic polishes but also fortifies your home against the harshness of chemical abrasives.

Embarking on this uncharted territory with castor oil is akin to discovering a hidden path in a welltrodden garden—a path that leads to innovation, sustainability, and a deeper appreciation for the versatility of natural products in our lives. This chapter is an invitation to view castor oil through a lens of creative possibilities, exploring practical yet innovative uses that showcase how traditional and modern practices can fuse, producing benefits that ripple through our lifestyles and into the environment.

5.1 ARTS AND CRAFTS WITH CASTOR OIL

In the eclectic world of arts and crafts, the fusion of functionality and creativity often births innovations that not only captivate the artistic mind but also echo sustainability. Among such innovations, castor oil emerges as an unexpectedly versatile medium, bridging traditional handicraft with contemporary ecofriendly practices.

Picture yourself immersed in the serene ambiance of your workshop, the air tinged with anticipation as you explore the tactile joys of your craft. Here, castor oil isn't just a background player; it becomes integral to the creation process, offering both substance and sustainability. Its utility in arts and crafts is as diverse as the palette of an artist, stretching across various textures and forms—from the simplest paper crafts to the complexities of fabric arts.

In Paper Mache and Sculptures

In the realm of paper mache, castor oil introduces a surprising element of durability. By incorporating it into the glue mixture typically used in paper mache, crafters find that their creations develop a harder, more resilient finish once dried. This is particularly advantageous for sculptors working on large installations or intricate pieces destined for outdoor display, where moisture and other elements might otherwise compromise the integrity of their artworks.

Fabric and Textile Innovation

The versatility of castor oil extends into textiles, where it serves as a softening agent in fabric dyes. Artists and designers dabbling in natural dyes can use castor oil to enhance the depth and richness of colors. The oil acts as a binding agent that helps the dye adhere better to the fabric, resulting in vibrant, longlasting hues. Moreover, in the world of fabric painting, castor oil mixed with pigments helps create a smooth application, preventing the harsh lines and drips that might mar the canvas.

In Woodworking and Furniture

Let's shift our focus to woodworking, where the protective qualities of castor oil are treasured. For the woodworker, the oil is a boon for treating wooden surfaces, providing a natural sheen that rivals any synthetic varnish. When mixed with natural resins, castor oil can be used to create a nontoxic wood finish that not only enhances the grain of the wood but also encapsulates the furniture piece with a durable protective layer against the wear and tear of daily use.

Crafting with Natural Fibers

Delving into crafting with natural fibers reveals yet another facet of castor oil's versatility. For those who spin yarn or work with felting techniques, castor oil can be used as a conditioning agent. Adding just a few drops into the fibers makes them easier to manipulate, reducing static and friction, which often frustrates artisans working with delicate or stubborn materials.

Art Preservation and Restoration

In the delicate realm of art preservation, castor oil offers a gentle solution for cleaning and restoring old paintings and fabrics. Since it does not contain the harsh chemicals found in conventional cleaning agents, it is employed cautiously by conservators to revitalize aged canvases without risking damage to the underlying paint or fabric.

Candle Making and Wax Crafts

The journey through castroduction does not stop at visual arts; castor oil finds its significance in the art of candle making as well. Candle enthusiasts experimenting with natural waxes like beeswax or soy wax use castor oil to achieve a smoother texture and a more consistent burn. Its addition to wax also aids in better scent retention and dispersion when essential oils are used, enhancing both the aesthetic and sensory experience of handmade candles.

Harnessing a NonToxic Approach

What stands out in each application—be it in sculpting, fabric arts, or candle making—is the consistent drive towards a nontoxic, sustainable approach to crafting. This is where castor oil truly shines, aligning with the modern crafter's desire to harmonize their creative expressions with environmental consciousness.

As we embrace these creative endeavors, castor oil serves not just as a tool, but as a gateway to rethinking how materials are used in art and craft. It encourages artists and crafters alike to consider the ecological footprint of their creations, promoting practices that support both the environment and the enduring beauty of their work.

By integrating castor oil into various mediums and techniques, what emerges is a tapestry of innovation that not only enhances the craft but also embeds sustainability into the very threads of artistic expression. Each stroke, each weave, each carvution is a testament to the possibilities that await when we dare to blend tradition with transformative, ecofriendly practices. In the grand canvas of arts and crafts, castor oil indeed sketches its legacy, one creation at a time, fostering a craft culture that values durability, beauty, and above all, sustainability.

5.2 Wellness Rituals and Ceremonies

In the serene realm of personal wellness, rituals and ceremonies occupy a place of profound significance. These practices, often steeped in ancient wisdom, bridge the gap between the physical and the spiritual, fostering a deep connection to oneself and the surrounding world.

Castor oil, with its rich history and multifarious benefits, has emerged as a compelling element in such rituals, enhancing their essence and effectiveness.

Imagine entering a space, be it a corner of your home or a more formal setting, where the air is infused with tranquility and the subtle, earthy scent of castor oil. This scenario sets the stage for a wellness ritual that not only soothes the body but also calms the mind and nurtures the soul. The integration of castor oil into wellness rituals is not just about harnessing its physical healing properties; it is about crafting a holistic ritualistic experience that resonates on multiple levels of being.

Rituals for Body and Mind

In many cultures, the act of massage is not merely physical therapy; it's a form of ritual that restores balance and harmony within the body. Castor oil, known for its antiinflammatory and moisturizing properties, is particularly suited for this purpose. Envision a ritual where warm castor oil, perhaps blended with essences like lavender or chamomile, is massaged into the skin. This not only stimulates the body's lymphatic system but also promotes relaxation, helping to release the stresses of the day.

Ceremonies to Honor the Self and Nature

Transitioning from personal wellness rituals to ceremonies that honor the broader aspects of life and nature, castor oil can play a pivotal role. For instance, consider a ceremony designed to mark the change of seasons—a time to acknowledge the cyclic nature of life and our place within these rhythms. Here, castorial might be used to light lamps or candles, symbolizing the light that guides us through seasonal transitions, illuminating paths and warming spirits as the earth cycles through its phases.

Meditative Practices Enhanced with Castor Oil

The incorporation of castor oil into meditative practices can greatly enhance the sensory experience, facilitating deeper states of relaxation and introspection. A few drops of warm castor oil applied to the forehead or feet before meditation can help stabilize and ground the practitioner, making it easier to journey inward. The oil's texture and warmth add a layer of comfort, distancing distractions and fostering a conducive environment for meditation.

Enhanced Healing Ceremonies

In therapeutic settings, ceremonies employing castor oil packs on specific areas of the body can be a powerful tool for healing. This traditional remedy, often placed over the abdomen, leverages the oil's potential to improve circulation and promote healing from within. Such ceremonies might include guided visualization or chanting, practices that complement the physical aspects of the oil treatment, invoking a holistic healing experience that addresses both emotional and physical ailments.

Rituals of Purification

Another profound utilisation of castor oil is in rituals of purification. In various traditions, castorial is employed in the cleaning of sacred spaces, purifying them before important rituals. This practice not only cleanses physical spaces but also metaphorically "clears the air," setting a pristine, sanctified tone that honors the sacredness of ritual activities.

Community Healing and Bonding

On a communal level, castor oil can facilitate rituals that foster group bonding and collective healing. One might imagine a community gathering where each participant receives a small amount of castor oil to rub into their hands. As they do so, they focus on their intentions for the gathering, infusing the oil with their thoughts and energies before jointly applying it in a communal healing ritual. This collective application, accompanied by shared prayers or intentions, weaves individual energies into a tapestry of communal support and wellbeing.

Connecting with Traditional Roots

For many, integrating castor oil into rituals and ceremonies is also a way of connecting with ancestral wisdom and practices. This retracing of traditional uses invites a deeper understanding of how such rituals have supported human health and spiritual wellbeing through the ages. It is an exploration of how ancient practices can be revitalized and adapted to serve contemporary needs, enriching our modern lives with the wisdom of the past.

Throughout all these applications, the key is the intentional use of castor oil as a medium for transferring energy, intention, and healing. It is a substance that, while simple in essence, performs complex roles in the rituals and ceremonies designed to enrich and beautify human life. Each drop of castor oil used ceremonially is imbued with intentions, and its application becomes a sacred act, a deep communion with the self and the universe.

Through such practices, castor oil transcends its physical properties, becoming a vessel for deeper spiritual exploration and holistic wellbeing.

5.3 LIFESTYLE INTEGRATION TIPS

In the tapestry of daily life, integrating natural elements can transform routine into ritual, turning the mundane into something magical. Castor oil, an unassuming yet potent elixir, offers just this kind of transformation. Its integration into daily practices does more than harness health benefits; it fosters a deeper connection to natural wellness and sustainable living. Here we explore ways to weave castor oil into the fabric of everyday life, enriching routines with its therapeutic and ecological virtues.

Imagine starting the day with castor oil as a cornerstone of morning wellness rituals. For many, mornings begin with skincare routines that set the tone for the day. Incorporating castor oil as a natural moisturizer can not only enhance skin health but also provide a moment of selfcare that grounds and centers the user before the day unfolds. Beyond its hydrating properties, the routine of applying castor oil is a tactile reminder of the body's needs for care and attention, creating a daily ritual that emphasizes mindfulness and selfcompassion.

Moving through the day, castor oil can continue to play a subtle yet powerful role. For those who spend hours at a desk, intermittent applications of castor oil to the wrists or temples can rejuvenate the senses and help maintain focus. Its soothing properties can also make it a wonderful stress reliever; a small dab rubbed between palms inhaling deeply gives a brief but potent sensory escape, reenergizing the mind and body.

In the home, castor oil takes on a different role as a tool for creating a healthier living environment. Its use as a natural cleaner, for instance, transforms cleaning from a chore into an act of caring for the health of one's family and the planet. Adding castor oil to homemade cleaning solutions not only effectively cleans surfaces but also avoids the toxins often found in commercial products, making the home a safer, more sustainable place.

The kitchen, too, can benefit from the inclusion of castaronil. As a natural preservative, a thin layer of castor oil applied to kitchen tools and appliances can help protect them from rust and wear. This practice not only extends the life of these tools, promoting sustainability, but also imbues routine maintenance with a sense of purpose and care, emphasizing the value of preserving rather than discarding.

At day's end, castor oil can transform bedtime routines into soothing rituals that promote quality sleep and relaxation.

A castor oil pack, placed on the abdomen or tired muscles, can ease tension and foster a sense of calm. Furthermore, integrating castor oil into nighttime skincare routines can rejuvenate the skin, locking in moisture and nutrients while the body rests.

Seasonal rituals also provide opportunities for integrating castor oil into life. In winter, using castor oil in homemade lip balms or hand creams can combat dry, harsh conditions, offering a sensory reminder of summer's warmth. During the warmer months, a light castor oilbased lotion can soothe sunexposed skin, seamlessly fitting into summer skincare rituals.

Family activities offer yet another venue for integrating castor oil into daily life. Crafting projects that use castor oil, whether in making simple candles, soaps, or other crafts, not only provide practical outcomes but also teach valuable lessons about selfsufficiency and the importance of natural ingredients. These activities, shared among family members, become cherished rituals that bond, teach, and entertain.

For those who travel, bringing along castor oil can ensure that the benefits of natural selfcare continue while away from home. Its compact versatility means that it can serve multiple purposes, reducing the need for numerous products. Its use as a quick cleanscape, makeup remover, or protective hair coat is invaluable, making it a staple in any travel kit.

Behind each of these applications is a shared principle: that integrating natural practices like those involving castor oil into everyday life can elevate our routines and help us live more consciously and harmoniously with nature. The rituals we cultivate, small as they may seem, can have profound effects on our wellbeing and the health of our environment.

In embracing castor oil as a multifaceted tool, we open up a world where daily routines become enriching rituals, where every application is an opportunity to connect with the essence of natural wellness. It's in these small moments that we find the true beauty of integrating castor oil into our lives—not merely for its physical benefits but for its ability to enrich, soothe, and simplify. Through these practices, we craft a life that not only nourishes the body but also feeds the soul.

www.ingramcontent.com/pod-product-compliance
Lightning Source LLC
Chambersburg PA
CBHW081547250726
48653CB00009B/3313